BOTTOM LINE'S GUIDE TO
Healing Foods

What to eat to BEAT heart disease, diabetes, cancer, dementia, pain and more!

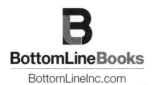

BottomLineBooks
BottomLineInc.com

Bottom Line's Guide to Healing Foods

Copyright © 2018 by Bottom Line Inc.

10 9 8 7 6 5 4 3 2 1

ISBN 0-88723-796-7

Bottom Line Books® publishes the advice of expert authorities in many fields. These opinions may at times conflict as there are often different approaches to solving problems. The use of this material is no substitute for health, legal, accounting or other professional services. Consult competent professionals for answers to your specific questions.

Telephone numbers, addresses, prices, offers and websites listed in this book are accurate at the time of publication, but they are subject to frequent change.

Bottom Line Books® is a registered trademark of Bottom Line Inc.,
3 Landmark Square, Suite 201, Stamford, CT 06901

BottomLineInc.com

Bottom Line Books® is an imprint of Bottom Line Inc., publisher of print periodicals, e-letters and books. We are dedicated to bringing you the best information from the most knowledgeable sources in the world. Our goal is to help you gain greater wealth, better health, more wisdom, extra time and increased happiness.

Printed in the United States of America

Contents

2. SUPERFOODS THAT SAVE YOUR EYES

3. SUPERFOODS THAT FIGHT CANCER

4. SUPERFOODS TO FIGHT ALLERGIES AND RESPIRATORY CONDITIONS

5. SUPERFOODS THAT HELP YOUR BRAIN

CHAPTER 1

Superfoods for Your Heart

Five Foods Proven to Prevent Heart Attacks

Bonnie T. Jortberg, RD, CDE, senior instructor, department of family medicine at University of Colorado at Denver and Health Sciences Center. She is coauthor of *The Step Diet Book.*

C ardiovascular disease is still the number-one killer in America. It accounts for about 37% of all deaths, according to the American Heart Association. Most of us know that a diet rich in fruits, vegetables and whole grains and low in saturated animal fats lowers the risk of heart disease. But certain foods have been shown to be particularly beneficial. Of course, no food is a magic bullet—you still need to exercise daily and maintain a healthy weight—but eating the recommended amounts of the following can go a long way toward preventing heart disease...

Spinach

Like most fruits and vegetables, spinach is rich in vitamins and minerals. What makes spinach stand out for keeping the heart healthy is folate, one of the B vitamins. According to several studies, including an extensive report from the Harvard School of Public Health, folate helps prevent the buildup of homocysteine, an amino acid in the blood that is a major risk factor for heart disease and stroke.

How much: Two cups of raw spinach (about two ounces) has 30% of the daily value (DV) for folate...one-half cup of cooked spinach provides 25%. Frozen and fresh spinach are both good, but beware of canned spinach—it may have excessive amounts of salt. Too much salt increases blood pressure, and high blood pressure is another major risk factor for cardiovascular disease.

Alternatives: Asparagus. Four spears have 20% of the DV of folate. Also, many breakfast cereals are fortified with folate—check the labels.

Salmon

Salmon is rich in omega-3 fatty acids. Omega-3s reduce inflammation and make your blood less "sticky," which prevents plaque—fatty deposits—from clogging your arteries. Having unclogged arteries reduces the risk of heart attack and stroke.

How much: The American Heart Association recommends two to three three-ounce servings of salmon a week. Fresh or frozen, farmed or wild, is fine, but go easy on canned salmon, which may be high in salt.

Alternatives: Other cold-water fish high in omega-3 fatty acids include mackerel, lake trout, sardines, herring and albacore tuna. If you don't like fish, have one teaspoon of ground flaxseeds daily—sprinkle on cereal, yogurt or salads, and drink plenty of water to avoid constipation.

Tomatoes

Tomatoes are loaded with lycopene, a carotenoid that gives them their color. Lycopene reduces cholesterol in the body. Too much cholesterol can lead to atherosclerosis (hardening of the arteries), which decreases blood flow to the heart—and that can lead to heart attack and stroke.

Cooked and processed tomato products, such as spaghetti sauce and tomato juice, provide the greatest benefits. Researchers at Cornell University found that cooking or processing tomatoes boosts lycopene levels and makes lycopene easier for the body to absorb. Look for low-sodium or no-salt-added products.

If you like ketchup, another source of lycopene, buy an organic brand, made with pure cane sugar, not processed high-fructose corn syrup. Organic ketchup can contain up to three times as much lycopene as nonorganic brands, according to a study published by the United States Department of Agriculture. Other organic tomato products weren't studied, so it is not yet known if they're also higher in lycopene.

How much: One cup of tomato juice (about 23 milligrams, or mg, of lycopene) or one-half cup of tomato sauce (20 mg) daily. A medium raw tomato has 4.5 mg.

Alternative: Watermelon (one-and-a-half cups of cut-up watermelon contain 9 mg to 13 mg of lycopene).

Oatmeal

Oatmeal is one of the best and most-studied sources of soluble fiber. Soluble fiber absorbs water and turns to gel during digestion. It then acts like a sponge to absorb excess cholesterol from your body. That's good for your heart. Studies show that five grams (g) to 10 g of soluble fiber a day can reduce LDL "bad" cholesterol by about 5%.

Soluble fiber also helps remove saturated fat in your digestive tract before your body can absorb it. That's also good for your heart.

How much: One-and-a-half cups of cooked oatmeal daily. This provides 4.5 g of fiber, enough to lower cholesterol. Rolled oats and steel-cut oatmeal work equally well to help lower cholesterol, but beware of flavored instant oatmeal—it is likely to have sugar added. Too much sugar in your diet increases the chance of inflammation, a risk factor for atherosclerosis. Sugar also can lead to weight gain, which is another risk factor for cardiovascular disease.

Alternatives: Kidney beans and brussels sprouts each have three grams of soluble fiber per one-half cup cooked.

Pomegranates

Pomegranates are loaded with polyphenols, antioxidants that neutralize free radicals, which can damage the body's cells. Polyphenols help maintain cardiovascular health by scooping up free radicals before they damage arteries. They also are believed to reduce LDL "bad" cholesterol. Red wine and purple grape juice are great sources of polyphenols, but pomegranates have the highest amount.

How much: 1.5 ounces of concentrated pomegranate juice daily. This is the amount used in most studies. Look for products that are labeled 100% juice, or concentrated, with no added sugar.

Caution: Pomegranate juice may affect the metabolism of prescription drugs and may cause blood pressure to decrease too much when combined with certain blood pressure medications. Check with your doctor.

Alternatives: Red wine (no more than two five-ounce glasses a day for men and one for women) and purple grape juice (four to six ounces a day).

Six Tasty, Surprising Foods That Protect Your Heart

Janet Bond Brill, PhD, RDN, FAND, is a nutrition, health and fitness expert specializing in cardiovascular disease prevention. Dr. Brill is a columnist in *Bottom Line Health* newsletter and is the author of *Blood Pressure DOWN, Cholesterol DOWN* and *Prevent a Second Heart Attack.* DrJanet.com

Just about everyone knows that a Mediterranean-style diet can help prevent heart disease. Even if you've already had a heart attack, this style of eating—emphasizing such foods as fish and vegetables—can reduce the risk for a second heart attack by up to 70%.

Problem: About 80% of patients with heart disease quit following dietary advice within one year after their initial diagnosis. That's often because they want more choices but aren't sure which foods have been proven to work.

Solution: Whether you already have heart disease or want to prevent it, you can liven up your diet by trying foods that usually don't get much attention for their heart-protective benefits…

SECRET 1: **Popcorn.** It's more than just a snack. It's a whole grain that's high in cholesterol-lowering fiber. Surprisingly, popcorn contains more fiber, per ounce, than whole-wheat bread or brown rice.

Scientific evidence: Data from the 1999–2002 National Health and Nutrition Examination Survey found that people who eat popcorn daily get 22% more fiber than those who don't eat it.

Important: Eat "natural" popcorn, preferably air-popped or microwaved in a brown paper bag, without added oil. The commercially prepared popcorn packets generally contain too much salt, butter and other additives. Three cups of popped popcorn, which contain almost 6 g of fiber and 90 calories, is considered a serving of whole grains. Studies have shown that at least three servings of whole grains a day (other choices include oatmeal and brown rice) may help reduce the risk for heart disease, high cholesterol and obesity.

SECRET 2: **Chia seeds.** You're probably familiar with Chia pets—those terra-cotta figures that sprout thick layers of grassy "fur." The same seeds, native to Mexico and Guatemala, are increasingly available in health-food stores. I consider them a superfood because they have a nutrient profile that rivals heart-healthy flaxseed.

In fact, chia seeds contain more omega-3 fatty acids than flaxseed. Omega-3s increase the body's production of anti-inflammatory eicosanoids, hormone-like substances that help prevent "adhesion molecules" from causing plaque buildup and increasing atherosclerosis.

Scientific evidence: A study published in the *Journal of the American College of Cardiology*, which looked at nearly 40,000 participants, found that an omega-3 rich diet can prevent and even reverse existing cardiovascular disease.

Other benefits: One ounce of chia seeds has 10 g of fiber, 5 g of alpha-linolenic acid and 18% of the Recommended Dietary Allowance for calcium for adults ages 19 to 50.

Chia seeds look and taste something like poppy seeds. You can add them to baked goods, such as muffins, or sprinkle them on salads and oatmeal or other cereals.

SECRET 3: **Figs.** They're extraordinarily rich in antioxidants. And, fresh figs are among the best sources of beta-carotene and other heart-healthy carotenoids.

Scientific evidence: In a study published in the *Journal of the American College of Nutrition*, two groups of participants were "challenged" with sugary soft drinks, which are known to increase arterial oxidation. Oxidation in the arteries triggers atherosclerosis, a main risk factor for heart disease. Those who were given only soda had a drop in healthful antioxidant activity in the blood...those who were given figs as well as soda had an increase in blood antioxidant levels.

Bonus: Ten dried figs contain 140 mg of calcium. Other compounds in figs, such as quercetin, reduce inflammation and dilate the arteries. Perhaps for these reasons, people who eat figs regularly have much less heart disease than those who don't eat them, according to studies. Most dried figs contain added sulfites, so it's best to buy organic, sulfite-free dried figs.

SECRET 4: **Soy protein.** Tofu, soy milk and other soy foods are "complete proteins"—that is, they supply all of the essential amino acids that your body needs but without the cholesterol and large amount of saturated fat found in meat.

Scientific evidence: People who replace dairy or meat protein with soy will have an average drop in LDL "bad" cholesterol of 2% to 7%, according to research from the American Heart Association. Every 1% drop in LDL lowers heart disease risk about 2%.

A one-half cup serving of tofu provides 10 g of protein. An eight-ounce glass of soy milk gives about 7 g. Edamame (steamed or boiled green soybeans) has about 9 g per half cup. Avoid processed soy products, such as hydrogenated soybean oil (a trans fat), soy isoflavone powders and soy products with excess added sodium.

SECRET 5: Lentils. I call these "longevity legumes" because studies have shown that they can literally extend your life.

Best choices: **Brown or black lentils.**

Scientific evidence: In one study, published in the *Asia Pacific Journal of Clinical Nutrition*, the eating habits of five groups of older adults were compared. For every 20 g (a little less than three-fourths of an ounce) increase in the daily intake of lentils and/or other legumes, there was an 8% reduction in the risk of dying within seven years.

Lentils contain large amounts of fiber, plant protein and antioxidants along with folate, iron and magnesium—all of which are important for cardiovascular health.

Similarly, a Harvard study found that people who ate one serving of cooked beans (one-third cup) a day were 38% less likely to have a heart attack than those who ate beans less than once a month.

Caution: Beans have been shown to cause gout flare-ups in some people.

Important: Lentils cook much faster than other beans. They don't need presoaking. When simmered in water, they're ready in 20 to 30 minutes. You need about one-half cup of cooked lentils, beans or peas each day for heart health.

SECRET 6: Pinot Noir and Cabernet Sauvignon. All types of alcohol seem to have some heart-protective properties, but red wine offers the most.

Scientific evidence: People who drink alcohol regularly in moderation (one five-ounce glass of wine daily for women, and no more than two for men) have a 30% to 50% lower risk of dying from a heart attack than those who don't drink, according to research published in *Archives of Internal Medicine*.

Best choices: Pinot Noir, Cabernet Sauvignon and Tannat wines (made from Tannat red grapes). These wines have the highest concentrations of flavonoids, antioxidants that reduce arterial inflammation and inhibit the oxidation of LDL cholesterol. Oxidation is the process that makes cholesterol more likely to accumulate within artery walls.

Bonus: Red wines also contain resveratrol, a type of polyphenol that is thought to increase the synthesis of proteins that slow aging. Red wine has 10 times more polyphenols than white varieties.

In a four-year study of nearly 7,700 men and women nondrinkers, those who began to drink a moderate amount of red wine cut their risk for heart attack by 38% compared with nondrinkers.

If you are a nondrinker or currently drink less than the amounts described above, talk to your doctor before changing your alcohol intake. If you cannot drink alcohol, pomegranate or purple grape juice is a good alternative.

Chicory for Heart Health

Mao Shing Ni, LaC, DOM, PhD, a Santa Monica, California–based licensed acupuncturist and doctor of oriental medicine. He is cofounder of Yo San University, an accredited graduate school of Traditional Chinese Medicine in Los Angeles, and author of *Secrets of Longevity.* TaoOfWellness.com

Chicory, an herb that is popular in China and parts of Europe, contains a compound called inulin that helps strengthen the heart muscle—and may even be useful in treating congestive heart failure (a condition that causes inadequate pumping action of the heart).

One study found that chicory helps regulate an irregular heartbeat—a potentially dangerous condition that can lead to heart failure. Other research shows that chicory helps lower cholesterol levels and may slow the progression of hardening of the arteries.

My advice: In the US, chicory root is most often roasted for use as a brewed coffee substitute that can be found in most organic food markets. For heart health, drink one to two cups daily of chicory coffee substitute. Don't use chicory if you have gallstones or are allergic to plants in the ragweed family.

My favorite: Teeccino Mediterranean Java Herbal Coffee.

Radicchio, a type of leafy chicory, is also widely available. Eat it two to three times weekly (in salads, for example).

Five Foods That Fight High Blood Pressure

Janet Bond Brill, PhD, RDN, FAND, is a nutrition, health and fitness expert specializing in cardiovascular disease prevention. Dr. Brill is a columnist in *Bottom Line Health* newsletter and is the author of *Blood Pressure DOWN, Cholesterol DOWN* and *Prevent a Second Heart Attack.* DrJanet.com

Is your blood pressure on the high side? Your doctor might write a prescription when it creeps above 140/90—but you may be able to forgo medication. Lifestyle changes still are considered the best starting treatment for mild hypertension. These include not smoking, regular exercise and a healthy diet. *In addition to eating less salt, you want to consume potent pressure-lowering foods, including...*

Raisins

Raisins are basically dehydrated grapes, but they provide a much more concentrated dose of nutrients and fiber. They are high in potassium, with 220 milligrams (mg) in a small box (1.5 ounces). Potassium helps counteract the blood pressure-raising effects of salt. The more potassium we consume, the more sodium our bodies excrete. Researchers also speculate that the fiber and antioxidants in raisins change the biochemistry of blood vessels, making them more pliable—important for healthy blood pressure. Opt for dark raisins over light-colored ones because dark raisins have more catechins, a powerful type of antioxidant that can increase blood flow.

Researchers at Louisville Metabolic and Atherosclerosis Research Center compared people who snacked on raisins with those who ate other packaged snacks. Those in the raisin group had drops in systolic pressure (the top number) ranging from 4.8 points (after four weeks) to 10.2 points (after 12 weeks). Blood pressure barely budged in the no-raisin group. Some people worry about the sugar in raisins, but it is natural sugar (not added sugar) and will not adversely affect your health (though people with diabetes need to be cautious with portion sizes).

My advice: Aim to consume a few ounces of raisins every day. Prunes are an alternative.

Beets

Beets, too, are high in potassium, with about 519 mg per cup. They're delicious, easy to cook (see the tasty recipe on page 11) and very effective for lowering blood pressure.

A study at The London Medical School found that people who drank about eight ounces of beet juice averaged a 10-point drop in blood pressure during the next 24 hours. The blood pressure-lowering effect was most pronounced at three to six hours past drinking but remained lower for the entire 24 hours. Eating whole beets might be even better because you will get extra fiber.

Along with fiber and potassium, beets also are high in nitrate. The nitrate is converted first to nitrite in the blood, then to nitric oxide. Nitric oxide is a gas that relaxes blood vessel walls and lowers blood pressure.

My advice: Eat beets several times a week. Look for beets that are dark red. They contain more protective phytochemicals than the gold or white beets. Cooked spinach and kale are alternatives.

Dairy

In research involving nearly 45,000 people, researchers found that those who consumed low-fat "fluid" dairy foods, such as yogurt and low-fat milk, were 16% less likely to develop high blood pressure. Higher-fat forms of dairy, such as cheese and ice cream, had no blood pressure benefits. The study was published in *Journal of Human Hypertension.*

In another study, published in *The New England Journal of Medicine,* researchers found that people who included low-fat or fat-free dairy in a diet high in fruits and vegetables had double the blood pressure-lowering benefits of those who just ate the fruits and veggies.

Low-fat dairy is high in calcium, another blood pressure-lowering mineral that should be included in your diet. When you don't have enough calcium in your diet, a "calcium leak" occurs in your kidneys. This means that the kidneys excrete more calcium in the urine, disturbing the balance of mineral metabolism involved in blood pressure regulation.

My advice: Aim for at least one serving of low-fat or nonfat milk or yogurt every day. If you don't care for cow's milk or can't drink it, switch to fortified soy milk. It has just as much calcium and protein and also contains phytoestrogens, compounds that are good for the heart.

Flaxseed

Flaxseed contains alpha-linolenic acid (ALA), an omega-3 fatty acid that helps prevent heart and vascular disease. Flaxseed also contains magnesium. A shortage of magnesium in our diet throws off the balance of sodium, potassium and calcium, which causes the blood vessels to constrict.

Flaxseed also is high in flavonoids, the same antioxidants that have boosted the popularity of dark chocolate, kale and red wine. Flavonoids are bioactive chemicals that reduce inflammation throughout the body, including in the arteries. Arterial inflammation is thought to be the "trigger" that leads to high blood pressure, blood clots and heart attacks.

In a large-scale observational study linking dietary magnesium intake with better heart health and longevity, nearly 59,000 healthy Japanese people were followed for 15 years. The scientists found that the people with the highest dietary intake of magnesium had a 50% reduced risk for death from heart disease (heart attack and stroke). According to the researchers, magnesium's heart-healthy benefit is linked to its ability to improve blood pressure, suppress irregular heartbeats and inhibit inflammation.

My advice: Add one or two tablespoons of ground flaxseed to breakfast cereals. You also can sprinkle flaxseed on yogurt or whip it into a breakfast smoothie. Or try chia seeds.

Walnuts

Yale researchers found that people who ate two ounces of walnuts a day had improved blood flow and drops in blood pressure (a 3.5-point drop in systolic blood pressure and a 2.8-point drop in diastolic blood pressure). The mechanisms through which walnuts elicit a blood pressure-lowering response are believed to involve their high content of monounsaturated fatty acids, omega-3 ALA, magnesium and fiber, and their low levels of sodium and saturated fatty acids.

Bonus: Despite the reputation of nuts as a "fat snack," the people who ate them didn't gain weight.

The magnesium in walnuts is particularly important. It limits the amount of calcium that enters muscle cells inside artery walls. Ingesting the right amount of calcium (not too much and not too little) on a daily basis is essential for optimal blood pressure regulation. Magnesium regulates calcium's movement across the membranes of the smooth muscle cells, deep within the artery walls.

If your body doesn't have enough magnesium, too much calcium will enter the smooth muscle cells, which causes the arterial muscles to tighten, putting a squeeze on the arteries and raising blood pressure. Magnesium works like the popular calcium channel blockers, drugs that block entry of calcium into arterial walls, lowering blood pressure.

My advice: Eat two ounces of walnuts every day. Or choose other nuts such as almonds and pecans.

DR. JANET'S ROASTED RED BEETS WITH LEMON VINAIGRETTE

Beets are a delicious side dish when roasted, peeled and topped with a lemony vinaigrette and fresh parsley. This recipe is from my book *Prevent a Second Heart Attack*.

6 medium-sized beets, washed and trimmed of greens and roots

2 Tablespoons extra-virgin olive oil

2 teaspoons fresh lemon juice

1 garlic clove, peeled and minced

1 teaspoon Dijon mustard

¼ teaspoon kosher salt

¼ teaspoon freshly ground black pepper

¼ cup chopped fresh flat-leaf Italian parsley

Preheat the oven to 400°F. Spray a baking dish with nonstick cooking spray. Place the beets in the dish, and cover tightly with foil. Bake the beets for about one hour or until they are tender when pierced with a fork or thin knife. Remove from the oven, and allow to cool to the touch.

Meanwhile, in a small bowl, whisk together the olive oil, lemon juice, garlic, mustard, salt and pepper for the dressing. When the beets are cool enough to handle, peel and slice the beets, arranging the slices on a platter. Drizzle with vinaigrette, and garnish with parsley. Serves six.

The Truth About Yogurt: Don't Be Fooled By These Misconceptions

Leslie Bonci, RD, CSSD, MPH, owner of the Pittsburgh-based nutrition consulting company Active Eating Advice by Leslie. The former director of sports nutrition for the University of Pittsburgh Medical Center, Bonci is the author of numerous books, including *The Active Calorie Diet* and the *American Dietetic Association Guide to Better Digestion*.

Yogurt has long been a favorite of Europeans, but this creamy treat is now a staple in more American households than ever before.

Trap to watch out for: With yogurt's increasing popularity in the US, consumers must now be alert for trumped-up claims about the food's healthfulness.

It's true that researchers are uncovering more and more reasons to consume yogurt. For example, a study recently presented at a meeting of the American Heart Association found that women who consumed five or more servings of yogurt weekly lowered their risk of developing high blood pressure by 20% compared with those who ate one serving of yogurt per month.

But anyone who has shopped for yogurt recently knows that the dairy aisle is chock-full of options ranging from Greek yogurt and "yogurt-style" drinks like kefir to coconut and soy yogurts—and even "desserty" yogurts with candy toppings. So how do you know what to believe about all these products? Beware of these misconceptions...

MISCONCEPTION #1: Greek yogurt is always healthier than regular yogurt. Yogurt is produced by the bacterial fermentation of milk (usually cow's milk). Greek yogurt takes it a step further by straining out whey (the watery part of milk) and lactose (milk sugar) so that the result is a thick, creamy texture not unlike sour cream.

For the same amount of calories, most Greek yogurt has about twice the protein of regular yogurt...and less carbohydrates, sugar and sodium. Greek yogurt, however, has more saturated fat than regular yogurt. (For more on saturated fat, see below.) With regular yogurt, you also get more bone-strengthening calcium, which is partially lost from Greek yogurt when the whey is strained out.

Important: Even though Greek yogurt's processing leaves it with less sugar to start with, some products still add in generous amounts of sugary flavoring. For example, plain, unsweetened Greek yogurt typically contains about 6 g of sugar per eight-ounce serving—thanks to the remaining naturally occurring lactose sugar. When you see a Greek yogurt with 20 g or 25 g of sugar per serving, that means extra sugar has been added, typically in the form of honey or fruit purée.

Best bet: Buy plain yogurt (Greek or regular), and mix in fresh fruit—you'll get an extra serving of produce without all the sugar of a purée. If you like crunch, sprinkle in some seeds (sunflower and pumpkin work well) or nuts (like pistachios). Check labels for sneaky sugar aliases like "evaporated cane juice," date or coconut sugar and high-fructose corn syrup (HFCS).

MISCONCEPTION #2: Low-fat yogurt is a better choice than full fat. A 2015 *American Journal of Clinical Nutrition* study made headlines when researchers found that people who ate the most high-fat dairy products had lower rates of type 2 diabetes.

As it turns out, it's not the amount of fat we consume but the type that's important. Full-fat yogurt is high not only in saturated fat but also in conjugated linoleic acid, which may have a protective effect against type 2 diabetes. Also, the full-fat yogurt's rich, thick mouthfeel sends a message to the brain that says, "I'm satisfied. I don't need to keep eating." Once in the stomach, the fat takes time to digest and, as a result, you feel full longer.

So feel free to include a daily serving of full-fat yogurt, but balance it by cutting back on other forms of saturated fat, such as fried foods, meat, eggs and/or butter.

***MISCONCEPTION #3:* Yogurt has the most probiotics of all dairy.** Probiotics are "friendly" bacteria that can enhance digestion, relieve constipation and bloating and even improve immune functioning.

While yogurt usually contains a few strains of probiotics, kefir, which is similar to yogurt but drinkable and more tart, offers far more. In fact, some kefir products contain 10 to 12 strains of probiotics! Don't ditch your yogurt entirely, but go ahead and switch things up with some kefir. Try it in a smoothie, swirled in oatmeal or in hummus recipes.

***MISCONCEPTION #4:* People with lactose intolerance should avoid yogurt.** The good bacteria in both Greek and traditional yogurt actually predigest some of the lactose in dairy products, lessening the odds of troubling symptoms such as gas, bloating and diarrhea. (Greek yogurt is especially low in lactose due to the straining process.)

In fact, research suggests that these bacteria are so potent that the enhanced lactose digestion may last for weeks following regular consumption. However, the bacteria must be alive for this to happen, so be sure to select products with the words "live and active cultures" on the label.

Helpful: Start out eating only a couple of tablespoons and watch for gastrointestinal symptoms. If there are none, slowly increase your intake over a period of days.

Eat Foods That Fight Inflammation

Inflammation is linked to heart disease, diabetes, arthritis and cancer. *The following foods may reduce inflammation in the body:* **Cabbage**—the sulforaphane in this cruciferous vegetable wards off inflammation-related diseases, such as cancer...**artichokes**—the antioxidants in this cactus reduce cholesterol, boost immunity and prevent premature aging...**tart cherries**—anthocyanins and quercetin in tart cherries are natural inflammation fighters...**pistachios**—these have lutein, resveratrol and other antioxidants that fight free-radical damage, and they have more cholesterol-lowering plant sterols than any other tree nuts...**onions**—sulfur compounds and quercetin in onions prevent inflammation and reduce blood pressure and cancer risk.

Best: Aim for at least one serving of one of these foods daily.

Jackie Newgent, RD, CDN, culinary and nutrition communications consultant, New York City, and author of *Big Green Cookbook: Hundreds of Planet-Pleasing Recipes & Tips for a Luscious, Low-Carbon Lifestyle.* JackieNewgent.com

If you still cannot tolerate dairy, there are non-milk-based yogurts, such as soy and coconut. But be aware that they don't have nearly as much protein as Greek yogurt and can be high in sugar (natural and/or added).

Coconut yogurt, with about 4 g of saturated fat per one-half cup, contains fats called medium-chain triglycerides—research suggests that the body may prefer to use these fats for energy versus storing them as fat.

MISCONCEPTION #5: **Yogurt is just a breakfast food.** With the right mix-ins, yogurt (Greek or regular) is a delicious treat any time of day.

To use plain yogurt: Make a higher-protein version of Brie or Rondelé cheese by emptying a large container of unflavored Greek yogurt into a strainer lined with a coffee filter and set over a bowl. Let it drain, refrigerate overnight, mix peppercorns and chives into the resulting yogurt "cheese" and use it as a spread with whole-grain crackers and crudités...or as a higher-protein cream cheese substitute.

Plain (regular) yogurt has a runnier consistency—use it to lighten up mac and cheese, mashed potatoes or your favorite stroganoff recipe (just cut back a bit on the milk, butter and cream, respectively).

For an indulgent-feeling, lower-calorie dessert, top one-half cup of full-fat vanilla Greek yogurt with one-quarter cup of chopped strawberries and a drizzle of chocolate balsamic vinegar. At just 130 calories and 11 g of sugar, this is a refreshing treat with an intense, not-too-sweet flavor.

18 Delicious Ways to Enjoy Heart-Healthy Walnuts

Debby Maugans, food writer based in Asheville, North Carolina, and author of *Small Batch Baking, Small Batch Baking for Chocolate Lovers* and *Farmer and Chef Asheville.*

Eating walnuts must be the tastiest way to protect your heart and your mind. Just a handful lowers "bad" LDL cholesterol and improves the way your blood vessels function. They're rich in alpha-linolenic acid, a plant form of omega-3 fat linked with better brain function and positive moods. And even though they are high in fat and calories, research finds that people who eat them regularly don't gain weight.

Our guess: It's because they are so satisfying. At 185 calories, a daily one-ounce serving (about seven halves, or one-quarter cup) provides heart-healthy benefits without derailing your diet.

Here are three recipes to try: Walnut Butter, Walnut Baba Ghanoush and Maple-Candied Walnuts (yes, healthful "candy!"). And see the tips at the end of this article to learn 15 more ways to enjoy walnuts.

Even Better Than Peanut Butter

WALNUT BUTTER

This one is so delicious that it can entice even the most resolute peanut butter devotee. We tested several versions using raw walnuts, toasted walnuts, nuts with a little olive oil to make it creamier, salt and no salt. The winner was a mixture of raw and toasted walnuts, a little salt and a teaspoon of honey to smooth out any residual bitter taste from tannins in traces of walnut peel that may cling to the nut after shelling. Toasting the walnuts adds texture and aroma, too.

Makes about one cup
2 cups chopped raw walnuts
1 teaspoon honey
¼ teaspoon salt
Preheat oven to 350° F.

Spread one cup of the walnuts on a baking sheet and bake until fragrant, 8 to 10 minutes. Let cool completely.

Place remaining raw nuts and the toasted/cooled walnuts in a food processor. Process until the mixture is a coarse paste, about 30 seconds. Add honey and salt, and process until smooth, 20 to 30 additional seconds. Scrape bowl as needed.

Store in a covered jar in the refrigerator.

A Nutty Twist to Eggplant Spread

WALNUT BABA GHANOUSH

For these flavors to blend and develop a richer overall flavor, refrigerate the dip for 4 to 6 hours. Remove from the refrigerator 30 minutes before serving.

Makes 1⅓ cups
1 (1- to 1¼-pound) eggplant, unpeeled

3 large shallots

Vegetable cooking spray

3 Tablespoons Walnut Butter (see recipe above)

1 Tablespoon fresh lemon juice

½ teaspoon salt

¼ cup crushed raw walnuts

Preheat oven to 400° F.

Remove stem end from eggplant, and cut in half lengthwise. Peel shallots and cut lengthwise into quarters. Place eggplant halves on baking sheet, cut sides up, and coat with cooking spray. Place shallots on baking sheet, and coat with cooking spray. Bake, turning shallots occasionally, until eggplant is very tender when pierced with fork and shallots are golden—about 45 to 50 minutes. Let cool on baking sheet.

Remove peel from eggplant and chop coarsely. Add to food processor with shallots, walnut butter, lemon juice and salt, then process until smooth, scraping bowl as necessary. Add walnuts and pulse until well blended, 2 or 3 times.

Transfer to a bowl, cover and refrigerate 4 to 6 hours. Remove from refrigerator 30 minutes before serving with crackers, pita bread or vegetables.

A Less Sweet Treat

MAPLE-CANDIED WALNUTS

Store-bought candied nuts often are coated with loads of sugar. A little pure maple syrup gives our candied walnuts just the right amount of sweet flavor with a crunchy crystal coating.

Makes 1 cup

1 cup raw walnut halves

2 Tablespoons maple syrup

⅛ teaspoon salt

Place a dry medium-size skillet on medium heat. When it is hot, and working quickly, add walnuts, maple syrup and salt. Stir until nuts are coated and let it cook, stirring frequently, until walnuts are toasted and syrup is almost evaporated but not burned.

Scrape out onto a sheet of wax paper, and let cool. As they cool, separate walnuts with a fork. Store in an airtight container. Eat as a snack...or use as a topping, such as over yogurt, oatmeal or salad.

15 More Ways to Enjoy Walnuts

The best way to have the freshest walnuts is to purchase them in their shells and open them as needed. The next best way is to purchase shelled walnut halves—they'll stay fresh longer than pieces. Store in a cool, dry place in an airtight container.

If the appearance in a recipe is important, you can dice them. When a recipe calls for crushed walnuts, place walnut halves in a freezer ziplock bag and roll with a rolling pin to crush them. You'll end up with pieces that appear almost ground and some that are finely broken.

Here are more tasty ways to slip walnuts into your diet...

1. When making a smoothie, toss in one-quarter cup of walnuts or two tablespoons of walnut butter.

2. Make a savory Walnut Crumble Topping to sprinkle on and season cooked vegetables. Mix one cup finely chopped, toasted walnuts, one cup whole wheat panko, one tablespoon minced fresh thyme, ⅛ teaspoon salt and one tablespoon extra virgin olive oil. Store in a sealed freezer bag in the freezer.

3. Sprinkle two tablespoons of finely chopped Maple-Candied Walnuts over a dish of yogurt or fruit for a naturally sweet dessert, snack or breakfast.

4. Make this appetizer: Stuff one-half teaspoon of goat cheese into a date, then tuck in a walnut half.

5. Before roasting fish fillets, coat them with crushed walnuts.

6. Grill or roast peach or pear halves. Drizzle one teaspoon of honey into each half and add one tablespoon of walnuts.

7. Make a kale salad with diced fresh pears and walnuts. Toss with vinaigrette.

8. Toss shaved and blanched brussels sprouts with a walnut vinaigrette. Crush ¼ cup walnuts. Sauté one minced shallot in two teaspoons walnut or olive oil. Add three tablespoons rice wine vinegar or Champagne vinegar and one teaspoon Dijon mustard in a small bowl. Stir in walnuts.

9. Add walnuts to brown rice to augment the protein in vegetarian main dishes.

10. For a heart-healthy dessert, dip walnut halves in melted dark chocolate and let them cool and harden.

11. Sprinkle crushed walnuts over mashed cauliflower. (No really—try it!)

12. Make a breakfast bowl of cooked oatmeal topped with chopped walnuts and vanilla yogurt.

13. Keep a jar of walnuts on your desk to snack on throughout the day.

14. Pack several single serving-size snack bags of walnuts mixed with dried cranberries (look for the kind that doesn't have added sugar) to keep handy for breakfast or lunch on the run.

15. Try walnut oil in salad dressings. It's made from nuts roasted before pressing, so it has a deep nutty flavor.

A Tasty Treat for Your Heart

Mark A. Stengler, NMD, a naturopathic doctor and founder of the Stengler Center for Integrative Medicine in Encinitas, California. He is author or coauthor of numerous books, including *The Natural Physician's Healing Therapies* and *Bottom Line's Prescription for Natural Cures*, and author of the newsletter *Health Revelations*. MarkStengler.com

We see headlines all the time that affirm the health benefits of chocolate. As a result, I see many people misinterpreting these headlines and eating way more chocolate than is good for them.

What a lot of these headlines don't tell you: Chocolate, as most of us know, is full of sugar and fat. Also, it is chocolate's main ingredient—cocoa—that is good for you. I want you to put down those commercially made chocolate bars and learn how to get the real health benefits of this incredible ingredient, even if you are a die-hard "chocoholic."

The first thing you need to know: The health claims are real. Recent research from the Karolinska Institute in Stockholm found that those who ate chocolate two or more times per week following a heart attack reduced their risk of dying from cardiovascular disease by 66%. And Spanish researchers recently found that consumption of chocolate reduced inflammation, a major component of many degenerative diseases.

The Best of Cocoa

Also known as cacao, the dried seed of the cacao tree is loaded with natural compounds called flavonoids, plant nutrients with antioxidant properties. The particular flavonoids found in cocoa are called flavanols—and they can prevent fatlike substances in the bloodstream from clogging your arteries. They have anti-inflammatory properties, and these flavanols help the body produce nitric oxide, a chemical that dilates and relaxes arteries, improving circulation and reducing blood pressure.

Best: Whenever possible, use organic raw cocoa powder as an ingredient in your recipes. It consists of 100% cocoa. Even though pure cocoa has a bitter taste, you need only use a small amount at a time to get the health benefits—and then the bitterness won't come through.

Examples: Add one to two tablespoons of cocoa powder to shakes and smoothies... or sprinkle it on fruit. Use it as a spice on vegetables and in salad dressings and soups. Of course, you can bake with it—and use it in a surprising variety of savory recipes, including chili, sauces and meat dishes. (See the Mexican Mole Sauce recipe on page 20.)

An OJ a Day Keeps the Cardiologist Away

Hesperidin, one of the main flavonoids found in citrus fruits, is believed to improve endothelial function—the ability of small blood vessels to expand, preventing arteries from clogging. Researchers at France's Centre de Clermont-Ferrand/Theix found that people who consumed hesperidin daily for one month (whether in orange juice or not) had better endothelial function than those who did not.

Recommended: One cup (eight ounces) of fresh OJ daily.

Mark A. Stengler, NMD, a naturopathic doctor and founder of the Stengler Center for Integrative Medicine in Encinitas, California. He is author or coauthor of numerous books, including *The Natural Physician's Healing Therapies* and *Bottom Line's Prescription for Natural Cures,* and author of the newsletter *Health Revelations.* MarkStengler.com

Several companies make excellent organic raw cocoa powder products. (Raw cocoa and cocoa powder are the same thing.)

Brands to try: Sunfood Cacao Powder, 16 ounces for $18.99 (888-729-3663, Sunfood.com) and Navitas Organics Cacao Powder, 16 ounces for $18.99 (888-645-4282, NavitasOrganics.com).

This type of cocoa is different from the type you buy in the baking section of the supermarket. Raw cocoa is cold-pressed (not cooked) to remove the fat. It provides more than three times as much antioxidant flavanols as cocoa that is made from fermented and roasted beans.

Second best: Know how to choose the most healthful chocolate bar. Organic dark chocolate—with a minimum of chemicals, processing and added sugar—is better for you than milk chocolate or white chocolate (which has no cocoa at all). Look for bars that have 60% to 85% cocoa. Choose those with the fewest ingredients. (Many chocolate bars have a host of unpronounceable ingredients and preservatives.) Choose bars with cocoa solids or cocoa mass (cocoa liquor) as the first ingredient, not sugar. Avoid those with milk, which negates the effects of the flavanols.

Brand to try: Scharffen Berger Extra Dark Chocolate or Bittersweet Dark Chocolate, $4.99 for a three-ounce bar (855-972-0511, Scharffenberger.com), available at specialty grocery stores, such as Whole Foods. Savor a square or two of high-quality chocolate several times a week (no more)—and you will safely reap the benefits of cocoa.

If You Are a "Chocoholic"...

For some people, eating chocolate can trigger addiction-like behavior. If you are one of those people who can't stop at one or two squares, it might be best to avoid chocolate bars altogether and instead use cocoa powder.

Cocoa for Dinner!

Jeannette Bessinger, CHHC, recipe designer for *The Healthiest Meals on Earth* and a chef/nutrition educator in Newport, Rhode Island, offers this savory recipe...

MEXICAN MOLE SAUCE FOR CHICKEN, TURKEY OR FISH

Serves 6 to 8

2 teaspoons olive oil

½ sweet onion, finely diced

1 clove garlic, minced

1 Tablespoon raw cocoa powder

1 teaspoon chili powder

1 teaspoon ground cumin

¼ teaspoon cinnamon

1 can (14-ounce) fire-roasted tomatoes, undrained

½–1 chipotle pepper in adobo (Spanish for "seasoning") sauce, diced, depending on how spicy you like it*

1 can (4-ounce) diced green chili peppers

¼ cup raisins

Heat the oil in a medium saucepan, and cook the onion until tender. Add the garlic and sauté. Stir in the cocoa powder, chili powder, cumin and cinnamon. Add the tomatoes, chipotle, green chilis and raisins. Bring to a boil, reduce heat, cover and simmer for 10 minutes. Cool slightly, and blend in a blender or food processor until smooth. It is spicy, so use sparingly.

*Most large grocery stores carry this canned sauce in the Mexican food section.

Pomegranate Juice and Your Heart

Mark A. Stengler, NMD, a naturopathic doctor and founder of the Stengler Center for Integrative Medicine in Encinitas, California. He is author or coauthor of numerous books, including *The Natural Physician's Healing Therapies* and *Bottom Line's Prescription for Natural Cures*, and author of the newsletter *Health Revelations*. MarkStengler.com

The pomegranate recently has been acclaimed for its health benefits. Pomegranate juice, which is available at health-food stores and most grocery stores, contains a blend of powerful, disease-fighting antioxidants, including phenolic compounds, tannins and anthocyanins.

Researchers in Norway found that pomegranates contain a higher concentration of antioxidants than 23 other fruits. This big red fruit has about 10 times more antioxidants than those with the next-highest levels, including grapes, oranges, plums, pineapples, lemons, dates, clementines and grapefruits.

Cleans Your Arteries

One of the major benefits of pomegranate juice is that it prevents the oxidation of "bad" low-density lipoprotein (LDL) cholesterol—a major cause of artery damage and subsequent plaque buildup.

For several years, Israeli researchers have studied the protective antioxidant and cardiovascular effects of pomegranate juice. In one of their most recent studies, pomegranate juice was found to reduce oxidation of LDL cholesterol by 40%. In another study, they found that pomegranate juice reduced the buildup of plaque in the carotid (neck) arteries, which supply blood to the brain.

Protects Diabetics' Arteries

Researchers from Shaheed Beheshti University of Medical Sciences in Tehran, Iran, found pomegranate juice to be helpful for people with diabetes. In this study, participants who consumed 40 g (about 1.4 ounces) daily of concentrated pomegranate juice for eight

A Delicious Daily Snack for Your Heart!

Here's a really heart-healthy snack —pomegranate juice and dates. It sounds like an odd random snack, but Israeli researchers report that in animal studies the combo reduced oxidative stress in the arterial walls by 33% while decreasing cholesterol by 28%.

In the study, they included antioxidant-rich date pits, which they ground into a paste. But even without the pits, the combination of juice and pitted dates is still superhealthy, according to the researchers. Their suggestion for people who want to protect their hearts—a daily snack of four ounces (one-half cup) of pure unsweetened pomegranate juice and three dates (also with no added sugar).

Study by researchers at Technicon-Israel Institute of Technology, led by Professor Michael Aviram of the Rappaport Faculty of Medicine and Rambam Medical Center, Haifa, Israel, published in *Food & Function*, a journal of The Royal Society of Chemistry.

weeks saw significant reductions in their total cholesterol and LDL cholesterol levels. This definitely is good news for diabetics because elevated blood glucose and insulin levels raise the risk of atherosclerosis.

I recommend that those with carotid stenosis (narrowing of the carotid arteries) and/or diabetes drink at least two ounces and up to eight ounces of 100% pomegranate juice daily. (Those with diabetes should drink no more than two ounces at a time, and take it with meals to slow down blood sugar absorption.)

For people trying to lower their blood pressure and those with a strong family history of heart disease, I recommend eight ounces a day.

You can, of course, dilute it by half with water (as I do) or combine it with other juices, such as grape or cranberry, for better flavor. One widely available brand that I use regularly is R.W. Knudsen Just Pomegranate.

Pomegranate supplements may prove to be a good alternative for people who wish to avoid the calories in pomegranate juice.

Awesome Avocados: Unique Ways to Enjoy This Heart-Healthy Dynamo

Janet Bond Brill, PhD, RDN, FAND, is a nutrition, health and fitness expert specializing in cardiovascular disease prevention. Dr. Brill is a columnist in *Bottom Line Health* newsletter and is the author of *Blood Pressure DOWN*, *Cholesterol DOWN* and *Prevent a Second Heart Attack*. DrJanet.com

With their silky texture, great flavor and numerous nutrients, you gotta love avocados! Technically a fruit, avocados are a potassium dynamo (one avocado contains more than twice as much blood pressure–lowering potassium as a banana). They also provide a variety of other minerals and vitamins, such as B vitamins, vitamin E and copper, and are packed with super-heart-healthy monounsaturated fat. If the only way you've ever eaten an avocado is sliced up in a salad or as guacamole, think again. These creamy gems are incredibly versatile and can be used in an array of tasty recipes. *Several different ways to use avocados plus some recipes to try…*

•**Grilled.** To grill an avocado, slice it in half, twist to pull apart and remove the pit, but leave the skin on. Brush the avocado flesh with a touch of extra-virgin olive oil and a spritz of fresh lime juice. Then place cut side down on a stovetop grill or an outdoor grill for five to seven minutes. Scoop out the flesh or serve in the skin as a tasty, warm side dish.

●**In a salsa.** Avocado salsa is a great topping.

To make: Toss one diced avocado with one diced fresh tomato and one-third cup of chopped red onion. Then drizzle with extra-virgin olive oil and fresh-squeezed lime juice, and season with salt and pepper. Spoon over your favorite grilled fish or a Mexican entrée.

●**As a substitute for mayo.** To replace artery-clogging saturated fat with a tasty healthy fat, try using ripe avocado in place of mayo on a sandwich or butter on bread. You can also make a heart-healthy green goddess salad dressing by using a ripe avocado instead of mayo and sour cream.

Ingredients:

1 cup of fresh spinach leaves

2 scallions

1 avocado

1 garlic clove

2 Tablespoons of white wine vinegar

2 Tablespoons of lemon juice

1 Tablespoon of olive oil

1 Tablespoon of fresh tarragon, chopped (or dried tarragon)

½ teaspoon of black pepper

What to do: Put all the ingredients in a food processor or blender and mix until smooth. It's a delicious dressing for potato salad or dip for veggies.

●**In ceviche.** This delicious, easy-to-make ceviche (a cold seafood dish) features two avocados plus cilantro for zest.

Ingredients:

1 pound of cooked shrimp (peeled, deveined and chopped)

2 avocados, chopped (about 1 cup)

½ red onion, chopped

¼ cup of fresh cilantro, minced

¼ cup of lime juice

½ teaspoon of ground black pepper

¼ teaspoon of salt

What to do: Mix all the ingredients together in a large bowl. Chill in the refrigerator for one hour. Serve with sliced bell peppers and/or cucumbers and pita chips or whole-wheat crackers.

Yield: 16 servings (1 serving = ⅛ cup).

•**In desserts.** Bet you didn't know that you can use avocado as a substitute for butter or oil in your favorite baked goods and desserts. One-half cup of puréed ripe avocado equals about one-half cup of butter. You can also use it to make a sinfully rich, heart-healthy dark-chocolate pudding.

Ingredients:

1 avocado

1 banana

⅓ cup of honey (or agave syrup)

⅓ cup of unsweetened, dark cocoa powder

¼ cup of peanut butter (or substitute any nut or seed butter)

What to do: Put all the ingredients in a food processor or blender and mix until the pudding is smooth.

Yield: 6 servings (1 serving = ⅓ cup).

Small Fish—Big Benefits!

Janet Bond Brill, PhD, RDN, FAND, is a nutrition, health and fitness expert specializing in cardiovascular disease prevention. Dr. Brill is a columnist in *Bottom Line Health* newsletter and is the author of *Blood Pressure DOWN, Cholesterol DOWN* and *Prevent a Second Heart Attack.* DrJanet.com

When it comes to fish that people either love or hate, sardines are among the top contenders. Iridescent and tiny, these oily fish within the herring family are oh, so flavorful when being enjoyed by their fans! But what if you can't imagine savoring sardines? Well, don't be so quick to swear off this miniature but mighty nutritional powerhouse. Keep reading, and you may just end up with an entirely new appreciation for this budget-friendly, convenient and superbly heart-healthy food.

Fresh sardines are tough to find and are highly perishable, so canned sardines are the go-to option for most people. Because canned sardines generally include the fishes' organs, skin and bones, they are a concentrated source of vitamins and minerals (especially calcium). You may already know that these petite fish are excellent sources of omega-3 fatty acids...are packed with vitamin D…and are rich in protein. But did you realize that one can (3.75 ounces) contains a whopping 1.4 g of heart-healthy omega-3 fat (that's about the same as a serving of sockeye salmon or tuna!) and 23 g of lean protein? Available just about anywhere (even at some gas stations and convenience stores), a can of sardines will cost you a paltry $3.50 or even less on sale.

And if that's not enough, consider this: Sardines are very low in heavy metal contaminants such as mercury—they feed on plankton, ranking them very low on the aquatic food chain.

The only bad news is that sardines from certain areas have been overfished and, as a result, appear on the "Avoid" list at SeafoodWatch.org, created by the Monterey Bay Aquarium, a nonprofit educational group that makes science-based recommendations for seafood sustainability. Since 2007, the Pacific sardine population has plunged by 90%—a decline that is believed to have contributed to the deaths of sea lions and brown pelicans across the West Coast. As a result, federal fishery managers have banned nearly all sardine fishing off the West Coast for the past several years. You can find sources of approved sardines from areas not affected by overfishing—they are certified by the Marine Stewardship Council (MSC), MSC.org, an international nonprofit organization established to address the problem of unsustainable fishing and safeguard seafood supplies for the future.

When choosing canned sardines, check the package label. Buy the kind packed in water or extra-virgin olive oil (stay away from those packed in other oils or sugary tomato sauce) and look for the MSC certification. On the convenience scale, sardines rate high because they can be served straight out of the can (or mashed with mustard and onions for a quick and delicious spread on crackers). *You can also try my favorite serving suggestions…*

• **Broiled.** Place your drained can of sardines on a baking tin lined with aluminum foil. Season with a drizzle of extra-virgin olive oil and one-half teaspoon of a fresh herb (such as rosemary), a few capers, a fresh garlic clove (minced) and a spritz of fresh lemon juice. Broil for a few minutes and serve.

• **Sardine-lemon-garlic pasta.** Fry one can of sardines (chopped) with two cloves of fresh garlic, juice from half a lemon and one-half cup of bread crumbs in extra-virgin olive oil. Add your own tomato sauce to the pasta bowl along with the sardine mixture, parsley and fresh Parmesan. Delizioso!

Why Sardines Are So Healthy

Karen Collins, MS, RDN, registered dietitian nutritionist, syndicated columnist and nutrition adviser to the American Institute for Cancer Research. She was an expert reviewer for the Institute's international report, *Food, Nutrition, Physical Activity and the Prevention of Cancer: A Global Perspective.* KarenCollinsNutrition.com

What makes sardines the sea's superfood? Canned sardines have more omega-3 fatty acids than most fish. And because they're a small fish that's low on the food chain, they contain less mercury than many other fish. They're also inexpensive and are a sustainable source of protein. So why do Americans eat only minnow-size amounts?

Sardines are an oily fish, and oily fish can taste a little…well, fishy. You might prefer sardines that are lightly smoked or sardines nestled in mustard or tomato sauce. (Or try the delicious recipes on the previous page!)

Here, more on the health benefits of sardines…

Great for omega-3s: A recent report from the USDA concluded that 80% to 90% of Americans eat less than eight ounces of fish a week, the minimum recommended amount. This means that you're probably not getting enough omega-3s, beneficial fats that have been shown to reduce the risk for heart disease and that may protect against cancer, depression, rheumatoid arthritis and other serious conditions.

All cold-water fish provide omega-3s, but sardines are among the best. A four-ounce serving of sardines has about 1.1 to 1.6 grams. That's right up there with salmon (1.2 to 2.4 g depending on the salmon) and much higher than cod (0.2 g) or the most common types of tuna (0.3 g).

Your body needs these important types of fats. A study published in *Neurology* found that people who ate fish three or more times a week were about 26% less likely to have silent infarcts, damaged brain areas that can lead to dementia and stroke. Omega-3s have been found to reduce heart irregularities (arrhythmias) that can be deadly and even may provide some blood pressure control help. Some experts speculate that the anti-inflammatory effects of omega-3s could help prevent some cancers…and eating more fish can help people eat less red meat or processed meat, important for decreasing the risk for colorectal cancer.

Other health benefits: Sardines are high in protein, vitamin D and selenium—and sardines with bones give an extra shot of calcium. A three-ounce serving of bones-in sardines has as much calcium as a glass of milk.

Less mercury: Some people avoid seafood altogether because they're worried about mercury, a contaminant found in virtually all fish, including farmed fish.

Good news: Sardines are among the lowest-mercury fish in the sea. They do contain trace amounts, but that might be offset by their high selenium content. The research isn't conclusive, but it's possible that a high-selenium diet could reduce the risks of mercury, either by "binding up" the mineral or by reducing its oxidative effects.

The health benefits of sardines and other fish more than outweigh the potential downsides of mercury—so much so that the EPA's and FDA's recently revised guidelines encourage pregnant women and young children (who are particularly susceptible to mercury) to eat eight to 12 ounces of low-mercury fish a week.

Sweet Potato—A Real Superfood for Your Heart

Janet Bond Brill, PhD, RDN, FAND, is a nutrition, health and fitness expert specializing in cardiovascular disease prevention. Dr. Brill is a columnist in *Bottom Line Health* newsletter and is the author of *Blood Pressure DOWN, Cholesterol DOWN* and *Prevent a Second Heart Attack.* DrJanet.com

D on't judge a book by its cover." This well-worn aphorism certainly applies to veggies...especially the sweet potato. This starchy root vegetable is, to be honest, not the most attractive food—with its odd shape, imperfect skin and dusting of dirt. But don't let the appearance stop you from incorporating it into your meals. Chock-full of vital nutrients, including vitamin A, vitamin C, beta-carotene, potassium, folate, fiber, B vitamins and manganese, the sweet potato is one of the healthiest complex carbs around.

Sweet potato or yam? Before we get too far along, let's clear up this confusion about sweet potatoes versus yams.

Here's the truth: Even though they're both tuberous root veggies, a yam is not even botanically related to a sweet potato! Real yams are typically imported from the Caribbean and generally sold only in international food markets in the US. A true yam, which has white interior flesh, is starchier and drier and not nearly as tasty as a sweet potato. It's worth noting, though, that the veggies that are often mislabeled as yams are actually soft sweet potatoes. With their copper-colored skin and orangey flesh, this variety becomes fluffy and moist when cooked. So opt for this one if you want to bake it—and especially if you're looking for that classic roasted sweet potato with the crispy skin and sweet, orange flesh.

Sweet potatoes come in purple, too. Did you know that there's a variety of purple potato that is actually a sweet potato, too? Available commercially in the US for about 10 years now, it is packed with even more antioxidants than its orange cousin. The purple hue is a giveaway that this variety is filled with anthocyanins—the same phytochemicals found in blueberries—which are powerful antioxidant and anti-inflammatory compounds that fight such diseases as heart disease and diabetes. For this reason, it's a good idea to splurge on purple potatoes (they usually cost about twice as much as regular sweet potatoes) whenever possible in lieu of the less nutritious white-fleshed varieties. No matter what type of sweet potato you choose, it's fun to add them to your diet in new ways.

My favorite spud ideas: Cube potatoes, roast them and add to salads or even mac and cheese…bake, scoop out the insides and add to baked goods such as muffins or pancake mix. *Or try my sweet potato hummus recipe…*

SWEET POTATO HUMMUS

Change up your basic hummus by making it sweet…or spicy, depending on your taste preference. *Ingredients…*

1 medium sweet potato, washed

1 15-ounce can of garbanzo beans, rinsed, drained

2 Tablespoons of extra-virgin olive oil

1 Tablespoon of tahini (optional)

Sweet spices: 1 teaspoon of cinnamon and 1 teaspoon of pumpkin spice

Spicy spices: ½ teaspoon of cayenne pepper, ½ teaspoon of paprika and 1 teaspoon of cumin

Instructions: Preheat oven to 400°F. With a fork, poke holes in the sweet potato all over (both sides). Place the sweet potato on a baking sheet and bake for 45 to 60 minutes (until you can squeeze it). Once cooked, remove the skin and chop the potato into pieces. Add the chopped sweet potato and the other hummus ingredients into a blender, and mix until it makes a smooth consistency with no visible pieces of sweet potato. Add either sweet or spicy spices. Taste and add more spices, if needed. Then enjoy!

The Mediterranean Diet Protects Your Heart...Even If You Cheat

Study titled "Dietary patterns and the risk of major adverse cardiovascular events in a global study of high-risk patients with stable coronary heart disease" by researchers at Auckland City Hospital, New Zealand published in *European Heart Journal*.

When it comes to eating a healthy diet, nobody's perfect. You might think you eat a heart-healthy Mediterranean diet, for example, but it's more than likely that what you actually eat is a "cheat-and-allow" version.

That's the one where you eat plenty of vegetables, fruits, beans, nuts, whole grains, yogurt, fish and moderate amounts of alcohol...but also ice cream, chips and fries, and maybe the occasional hot dog or two.

Are you fooling yourself that "somewhat healthy" is still healthy? Or should you work hard to get those chips and dips out of your life for real?

That's exactly the question that a recent large-scale global study set out to investigate.

Your Cheatin' Heart Healthy Diet

Researchers asked 15,000 heart disease patients in 39 countries to fill out questionnaires about how often each week they ate certain foods associated with a Mediterranean diet such as vegetables, fruit, whole grains, fish and alcohol—as well as typical "Western" refined grains, sugary desserts, sweets, soda and deep-fried foods. The study was actually part of a clinical trial for a drug to treat atherosclerosis, funded by the manufacturer of the drug, but the focus was on nutrition.

No surprise: Those who ate Mediterranean-diet foods most frequently had the lowest incidence of heart attack, stroke or death during the nearly four years of the study— 7.3% vs. 10.8% for those who ate these foods least frequently.

Big surprise: Those who ate unhealthy Western-diet foods most frequently did not have an increase in cardiovascular risk.

How can that be? The working theory is that the protective effect of the healthy Mediterranean foods outweighed any harm from less healthy food.

Now, these results are not carte blanche to stuff yourself with donuts and French fries—which are definitely not health foods. But they are a clear message that eating some unhealthy food doesn't have to make you unhealthy—as long as you also include fruits, vegetables, fish and whole grains. Doesn't that make you feel better?

Berries Help Your Heart

Mark A. Stengler, NMD, a naturopathic doctor and founder of the Stengler Center for Integrative Medicine in Encinitas, California. He is author or coauthor of numerous books, including *The Natural Physician's Healing Therapies* and *Bottom Line's Prescription for Natural Cures*, and author of the newsletter *Health Revelations*. MarkStengler.com

Researchers from the National Public Health Institute in Helsinki, Finland, analyzed the effects of berry consumption on 72 men and women (average age 58) at risk for cardiovascular disease. One group consumed berries—bilberries, lingonberries or strawberries—each day, while a control group had none.

Results: After two months, HDL (good) cholesterol rose by 5.2% in the berry group, and systolic (top number) blood pressure dropped by as much as 7.3 points in those with the highest baseline readings—versus almost no change in the control group. The berry group experienced an 11% inhibition in platelet function, making blood less likely to form dangerous clots.

My view: Polyphenols are powerful antioxidants found in cocoa, red wine and tea. They reduce blood pressure and help keep blood thin (reducing stroke risk). Berries also contain polyphenols and vitamin C, folate, potassium and soluble fiber. I commonly suggest that my patients eat more berries, a healthy alternative to sugary snacks.

Snack on Nuts

A survey of 25 clinical trials published in *Archives of Internal Medicine* has found that eating 2.4 ounces (about one-half cup) daily of any kind of nuts can lower both total cholesterol and LDL (bad) cholesterol. Snack on nuts—but since they are high in calories, reduce your intake of other high-calorie foods and snacks.

Mark A. Stengler, NMD, is a naturopathic medical doctor and leading authority on the practice of alternative and integrated medicine. MarkStengler.com

Black Raspberries Love Your Heart

Study titled "Black Raspberry Extract Increased Circulating Endothelial Progenitor Cells and Improved Arterial Stiffness in Patients with Metabolic Syndrome: A Randomized Controlled Trial" by researchers at Korea University Anam Hospital and Gochang Black Raspberry Research Institute, both in Seoul, South Korea, published in *Journal of Medicinal Food*.

Stephen Dunfield, president of BerriHealth, Corvallis, Oregon, which specializes in quality black raspberry products. BerriHealth.com

John La Puma, MD, board-certified specialist in internal medicine and trained chef with a private nutritional medical practice in Santa Barbara, California, and cofounder of the popular video series ChefMD. He is author of *Refuel: A 24-Day Eating Plan to Shed Fat, Boost Testosterone, and Pump Up Strength and Stamina.* DrJohnLaPuma.com

Let us pause for a moment to savor the sweet and tart black raspberry (Rubus occidentalis). It's got amazing health benefits that you won't get from red raspberries—or blackberries.

This rare native American fruit's fleetingly brief season is just a few mid-summer weeks in many parts of the country. But there are ways you can still enjoy black raspberries year-round—and you'll definitely want to.

Here's why: Black raspberries have had a reputation for anticancer properties. Now we know they're really good for your heart, too.

Keeping Blood Vessels Flexible and Healthy

The study, from South Korea, looked at men and women with metabolic syndrome, a combination of risk factors such as high blood pressure, belly fat, low HDL levels and insulin resistance that greatly increases the risk for cardiovascular disease and diabetes. Some of them took 750 mg of black raspberry extract daily for 12 weeks while the others took inactive placebo pills.

Result: Those who consumed black raspberry extract had less arterial stiffness, a key contributor to cardiovascular disease risk.

The science behind the benefit: Those who took black raspberry produced more compounds that stimulate the regeneration of the cells lining the blood vessels, helping them function better.

Black Raspberry Power

What's so healthy about these berries? For one, they are extraordinarily rich in antioxidants, with 10 times the antioxidant power of most fruits and vegetables—a mere four berries carries the same punch as an entire three-and-a-half ounce serving of, say, spinach.

Foremost among these antioxidants are flavonoid pigments, which give the berries their dark color. These compounds have already been shown to help protect LDL cholesterol from oxidation, a key factor of heart disease. They play a key role in anticancer effects, too—in animal studies, black raspberry extract may slow or reverse the growth of breast, prostate, cervical, colon, oral and esophageal cancers and is now being studied in human clinical trials of colorectal, stomach, oral and prostate cancers as well for the management of inflammatory bowel disease (IBD).

One class of black raspberry flavonoid in particular, anthocyanins, has been shown to improve vision, lower blood pressure, enhance immunity and improve memory. Compared with red raspberries, black raspberries have seven times more anthocyanins per serving.

Black Raspberry Supplements

If you want to enjoy these health benefits the rest of the year, you can purchase whole freeze-dried black raspberry powder or a liquid extract. One company that makes it and supplies it to researchers in Japan and the US is BerriHealth, based in Corvallis, Oregon. The recommended serving size of its powder is one teaspoon (four grams), which is the equivalent of 20 fresh berries and has 15 calories. You can mix it in water or juice, add it as a topping to yogurt or blend it into smoothies.

How does that amount compare with what was used in the Korean study? It's not possible to make exact comparisons, because that study used a different method to make the extract. But that teaspoon with 20 berries likely represents more than what was used in the study, which was, roughly estimated, the equivalent of seven or eight berries, according to Steve Dunfield, president of BerriHealth.

Cancer research studies have used even larger amounts—as much as 50 grams of freeze-dried black raspberry powder, the equivalent of three cups of fresh black raspberries—about 250 berries.

How much should you take? It depends on why you're taking it. If the purpose is to treat a health condition—especially a serious condition such as cancer—you should work with your doctor to determine what's right for you.

If you just want to enjoy the healthful properties of this berry year-round, on the other hand, let food amounts be your guide. After all, that's what the powder is—it's just whole black raspberry, including the seeds, with nothing added. If you put a teaspoon of powder in your smoothie, that's 20 berries. A tablespoon? That's like putting 60 berries in your drink. All that adds are a few extra calories—specifically, 45.

One caveat: Be careful of many black raspberry capsules on the market. Often these capsules do not contain much black raspberry, and many lack authenticity. Best to stick with either freeze-dried powders made from authentic whole black raspberries or well-prepared liquid extracts. According to Bottom Line medical contributing editor Andrew Rubman, ND, the Eclectic Institute is another reputable supplier of real black raspberry products, including freeze-dried black raspberry powder in bulk or in capsules.

> **Flaxseed Lowers Cholesterol**
>
> An Iowa State University study found that men with high total cholesterol who consumed at least 150 milligrams of flaxseed lignans daily (about three tablespoons) experienced a nearly 10% decrease in cholesterol levels. More research is needed to determine why eating flaxseed did not change cholesterol levels in women.
>
> *Best:* Sprinkle ground flaxseed on cereal.
>
> Mark A. Stengler, NMD, is a naturopathic medical doctor and leading authority on the practice of alternative and integrated medicine. MarkStengler.com

Get 'Em Fresh...While You Can

Fresh black raspberries are in season primarily in July, so don't hesitate to make tracks to a grocery store or your local farmer's market. They're delicious eaten fresh out of hand, puréed, baked into pie (try two parts black raspberry to one-part blueberry or blackberry), blended into smoothies or preserved in jam. (How to tell the difference between blackberries and black raspberries? Easy—all raspberries have a hollow core.)

Are black raspberries superior to blackberries and red raspberries for the heart? "Neither has been tested against black raspberries for cardiovascular effects," commented food-as-medicine expert John La Puma, MD, who wasn't involved in the study. "But in general, the blacker the berry, the greater the antioxidant effect—and oxidation of LDL cholesterol starts cardiovascular disease."

His advice: "Eat the berry you have, and enjoy it. All of them taste better than prescription medicine!"

Yummy, Easy Garbanzo Recipe Is a Super Healer

Debby Maugans, food writer based in Asheville, North Carolina, and author of *Small Batch Baking, Small Batch Baking for Chocolate Lovers* and *Farmer and Chef Asheville.*

Whether you call it "en papillote" as the French do…or "al cartoccio" as Italians do…or cooking in parchment, as we Americans say, sealing a meal in food-safe paper packages and baking it in an oven is a quick, easy and an especially healthy way to cook. Cooking in a sealed pouch is an age-old method. In Malaysia, it's in banana leaves. In Latin American, steamed corn husks. In China, water lotus leaves. And so on.

Nutrients, especially water-soluble vitamins, stay sealed in. Flavors and aromas are intensified when foods, spices and herbs steam in their own juices with no added water. With little or no added sauces or fats needed, you save calories. It's quick—most foods cook in 20 minutes. Plus, the sealed packages look impressive when you plate each one, and they are fun to open.

Bonus: No cleanup!

While you can't cook everything in parchment, it's easy enough to be your go-to favorite cooking method. Here's a recipe to get you started—Garbanzo Vegetable Curry Packages. It's a flavorful curry that uses super-healthy garbanzo beans (chick peas), which are rich in phytochemicals that protect you against cancer…complex carbohydrates that keep your blood sugar steady… and protein and fiber to keep you feeling full longer. They also lower LDL cholesterol.

Here's the recipe…

GARBANZO VEGETABLE CURRY PARCHMENT PACKAGES

½ cup reduced-fat coconut milk

1 clove garlic, minced

2 teaspoons grated ginger

2 teaspoons curry powder

¼ teaspoon salt

¼ teaspoon freshly ground pepper

1 cup cooked brown rice

1 cup canned garbanzo beans, rinsed and drained

1 cup small cauliflowerets

1 cup diced zucchini

¾ cup drained chopped tomatoes

Toppings, optional: ¼ cup unsweetened flaked coconut, ¼ cup dry roasted peanuts, ¼ cup raisins

Preheat oven to 400°F.

Prepare the parchment: Cut two large pieces of parchment paper for baking (at least 15 inches x 20 inches). Cut out a large heart shape by folding the paper in half and tracing a half-heart, keeping the fold at the center of the heart. Place each cut-out heart, opened, on a separate baking sheet.

Next, combine coconut milk, garlic, ginger, curry powder, salt and pepper in a bowl and mix.

Spoon ½ cup cooked rice in the center of one half of each parchment heart, keeping it close to the fold. Top each mound of rice with one-half each of the beans, cauliflowerets, zucchini and tomatoes. Drizzle each mound with one-half of the coconut milk and spice mixture.

Seal the packages: Fold the other half of the parchment heart over the rice and beans mixture so that the edges line up with the bottom half. Beginning at the top of the heart, fold the edges over and make small, tight pleats, creasing them firmly. Finish by twisting the point at the end to seal.

Bake until puffed and browned, 18 to 20 minutes. Place on plates, and cut an "X" in the tops of each package. Peel back the pointed edges to open. Serve with unsweetened coconut flakes, dry roasted peanuts and raisins to sprinkle on top.

Makes 2 servings.

Eat Your Way to Low Cholesterol: Surprising Superfood Cuts Heart Attack Risk 35%

Kenneth H. Cooper, MD, MPH, founder of The Cooper Clinic and The Cooper Institute for Aerobics Research, both in Dallas. A leading expert on preventive medicine and the health benefits of exercise, he is author of *Controlling Cholesterol the Natural Way.* CooperAerobics.com

I f you have high cholesterol, your primary objective should be to find a way to lower it without drugs and their side effects. The good news is that just eating the right foods often can reduce cholesterol by 50 points or more.

Most people know to eat a low-fat diet, but there are certain foods that can help lower cholesterol that may surprise you...

Macadamia Nuts

Macadamia nuts are among the fattiest plant foods on the planet, about 76% total fat by weight. However, nearly all of the fat is monounsaturated. This type of fat is ideal because it lowers LDL (bad) cholesterol without depressing HDL (good) cholesterol.

A team at Hawaii University found that study participants who added macadamia nuts to their diets for just one month had total cholesterol levels of 191 mg/dL, compared with those eating the typical American diet (201 mg/dL). The greatest effect was on LDL cholesterol.

Macadamia nuts are higher than other nuts in monounsaturated fat, but all nuts are high in vitamin E, omega-3 fatty acids and other antioxidants. Data from the Harvard Nurses' Health Study found that people who ate at least five ounces of any kind of nut weekly were 35% less likely to suffer heart attacks than those who ate less than one ounce per month.

Caution: Moderation is important because nuts—macadamia nuts, in particular—are high in calories. Limit servings to between one and two ounces daily—about a small handful a day.

Rhubarb

Rhubarb is ideal for both digestive health and lowering cholesterol because it contains a mix of soluble (see "Oats" on page 38) and insoluble fibers.

A study reported in *Journal of the American College of Nutrition* found that participants who ate a little less than three ounces of rhubarb daily for four weeks had an average drop in LDL cholesterol of 9%.

This tart-tasting vegetable isn't only an ingredient in pies. You can cut and simmer the stalks and serve rhubarb as a nutritious side dish (add some low-calorie strawberry jam for a touch of sweetness).

Rice Bran

It's not as well-known for lowering cholesterol as oats and oat bran, but rice bran is just about as effective and some people enjoy it more. A six-week study at University of California, Davis Medical Center found that people who ate three ounces daily of a product with rice bran had drops in total cholesterol of 8.3% and a reduction in LDL of 13.7%.

You can buy rice bran in most supermarkets—it's prepared like oatmeal. Or you can try prepared rice-bran breakfast cereals, such as Quaker Rice Bran Cereal and Kenmei Rice Bran.

Red Yeast Rice

Made from a yeast that grows on rice, red yeast rice contains monacolins, compounds that inhibit the body's production of cholesterol.

One study found that people who took red yeast rice supplements and did nothing else had drops in LDL of 23%. When the supplements were combined with healthy lifestyle changes, their LDL dropped by about 42%.

Red yeast rice may be less likely than statins to cause the side effect myopathy (a painful muscle disease).

Recommended dose: 600 milligrams (mg), twice daily. It is available online and at health-food stores.

> ### Broccoli Benefit
>
> Broccoli boosts arterial health. Research funded by the British Heart Foundation found that the phytochemical sulforaphane in broccoli and other cruciferous vegetables, such as kale, cabbage and cauliflower, can activate a protein in the arteries that prevents inflammation and buildup of fatty plaque, both of which can lead to heart attack and stroke.
>
> *Best:* Eat one-half cup of a raw or lightly steamed cruciferous vegetable daily.
>
> Mark A. Stengler, NMD, is a naturopathic medical doctor and leading authority on the practice of alternative and integrated medicine. MarkStengler.com

Green Tea

Green tea is a concentrated source of polyphenols, which are among the most potent antioxidants. It can lower LDL cholesterol and prevent it from turning into plaque deposits in blood vessels. In one study, men who drank five cups of green tea daily had total cholesterol levels that were nine points lower than men who didn't drink green tea.

Three to five cups daily are probably optimal. Black tea also contains polyphenols but in lower concentrations than green tea.

Vitamins C and E

These vitamins help prevent cholesterol in the blood from oxidizing. Oxidized cholesterol is more likely to cling to artery walls and promote the development of atherosclerosis, the cause of most heart attacks.

I advise patients with high cholesterol to take at least 400 international units (IU) of d-alpha-tocopherol, the natural form of vitamin E, daily. You might need more if you engage in activities that increase oxidation, such as smoking.

For vitamin C, take 1,000 mg daily. People who get the most vitamin C are from 25% to 50% less likely to die from cardiovascular disease than those who get smaller amounts.

The Big Three

In addition to the above, some foods have long been known to reduce cholesterol, but they are so helpful that they bear repeating again...

• **Cholesterol-lowering margarines.** I use Benecol every day. It's a margarine that contains stanol esters, cholesterol-lowering compounds that are extracted from plants such as soy and pine trees. About 30 grams (g) of Benecol (the equivalent of about three to four pats of butter) daily will lower LDL by about 14%.

Similar products, such as Promise Buttery Spread, contain sterol esters. Like stanols, they help block the passage of cholesterol from the digestive tract into the bloodstream. We used to think that sterols weren't as effective as stanols for lowering cholesterol, but they appear to have comparable benefits.

• **Oats.** They are among the most potent nutraceuticals, natural foods with medicine-like properties. Both oat bran and oatmeal are high in soluble fiber. This type of fiber dissolves and forms a gel-like material in the intestine. The gel binds to cholesterol molecules, which prevents them from entering the bloodstream.

A Harvard study that analyzed the results of 67 scientific trials found that even a small amount of soluble fiber daily lowered total cholesterol by five points. People who eat a total of 7 g to 8 g of soluble fiber daily typically see drops of up to 10%. One-and-a-half cups of cooked oatmeal provides 6 g of fiber. If you don't like oatmeal, try homemade oat bran muffins. Soluble fiber also is found in such foods as kidney beans, apples, pears, barley and prunes.

Eat to Fight Gum Disease... Help Your Heart

Periodontal (gum) disease is the leading cause of tooth loss. Research shows that this infection and/or inflammation of the gums also can lead to heart disease.

Best food: Kefir. This fermented milk is high in calcium (good for tooth enamel). It also contains the beneficial probiotic organism Lactobacillus, which secretes hydrogen peroxide and other substances that help kill the bacteria that cause gum disease.

What to do: Drink kefir in place of regular milk. Two or more one-cup servings daily have been linked to a reduced risk for tooth loss.

Also helpful: Live-culture yogurt. Many brands contain the same strain of Lactobacillus that is in kefir.

David Grotto, RD, LDN, a registered dietitian and founder and president of Nutrition Housecall, LLC, a Chicago-based nutrition consulting firm. He is author of *The Best Things You Can Eat.* DavidGrotto.com

Also helpful: Psyllium, a grain that's used in some breakfast cereals, such as Kellogg's All-Bran Bran Buds, and in products such as Metamucil. As little as 3 g to 4 g of psyllium daily can lower LDL by up to 20%.

•**Fish.** People who eat two to three servings of fish a week will have significant drops in both LDL and triglycerides, another marker for cardiac risk. One large study found that people who ate fish as little as once a week reduced their risk for a sudden, fatal heart attack by 52%.

I eat salmon, tuna, herring and sardines. Other good sources of omega-3 fatty acids include walnuts, ground flaxseed, tofu and canola oil.

Fish-oil supplements may provide similar protection, but they are not as effective as the natural food, which contains other beneficial nutrients as well.

Orange Peel for Cholesterol

Mao Shing Ni, LaC, DOM, PhD, a Santa Monica, California–based licensed acupuncturist and doctor of oriental medicine. He is cofounder of Yo San University, an accredited graduate school of Traditional Chinese Medicine in Los Angeles, and author of *Secrets of Longevity*. TaoOfWellness.com

As we age, LDL "bad" cholesterol often accumulates in the arteries, leading to heart disease and stroke. Orange peel actually may lower cholesterol better than some medications, such as statin drugs, without the side effects.

Studies show that compounds called polymethoxylated flavones (PMFs), found in pigments of oranges and tangerines, can reduce bad cholesterol—without decreasing the level of HDL "good" cholesterol.

My advice: Grate or chop the peel of an orange or tangerine (preferably organic to avoid potentially toxic pesticides) and add to your sauce. If cooking a 12-ounce serving of meat or chicken, use the whole rind. As an alternative, use low-sugar marmalade, which contains orange rind, in your sauce.

CHAPTER 2

Superfoods That Save Your Eyes

Foods That Fight Vision Loss

Mark A. Stengler, NMD, a naturopathic doctor and founder of the Stengler Center for Integrative Medicine in Encinitas, California. He is author or coauthor of numerous books, including *The Natural Physician's Healing Therapies* and *Bottom Line's Prescription for Natural Cures*, and author of the newsletter *Health Revelations.* Mark Stengler.com

A study sponsored by the National Eye Institute examined the link between nutrients and age-related macular degeneration (AMD), a leading cause of vision loss in people over age 65.

Results: Among 4,519 adults ages 60 to 80, those whose diets were highest in the carotenoids lutein and zeaxanthin had a 35% lower risk for developing "wet" AMD (the most severe form) than those with the lowest intake.

My view: Wet AMD is difficult to treat, so prevention is key. Lutein and zeaxanthin may protect the macula (part of the retina) from damaging ultraviolet rays.

Self-defense: Eat at least one daily serving (two servings if over age 50) of eggs, kale, spinach, turnip greens, collard greens, romaine lettuce, broccoli, zucchini, peas or brussels sprouts.

Save Your Sight: Natural Ways to Fight Common Eye Problems

Jeffrey R. Anshel, OD, founder of the Ocular Nutrition Society and president of Corporate Vision Consulting, based in Encinitas, California, where he also has the private optometry practice E Street Eyes. He is author of *What You Must Know About Food and Supplements for Optimal Vision Care: Ocular Nutrition Handbook.* SmartMedicineFor YourEyes.com

Vision problems in the US have increased at alarming rates, including a 19% increase in cataracts and a 25% increase in macular degeneration since 2000.

Why the increase? Americans are living longer, and eyes with a lot of mileage are more likely to break down. But not getting the right nutrients plays a big role, too—and the right foods and supplements can make a big difference.

Of course, people with eye symptoms or a diagnosed eye disease should work closely with their doctors. I also recommend medical supervision for people who are taking multiple supplements.

But here are common eye problems and the foods and supplements that can fight them...

Dry Eyes

The eyes naturally get drier with age, but dry-eye syndrome—a chronic problem with the quantity and quality of tears—often is due to nutritional deficiencies. Poor nutrition can permit damaging free radicals to accumulate in the glands that produce tears.

What to do: Take one-half teaspoon of cod liver oil twice a week. It's an excellent source of DHA (docosahexaenoic acid, an omega-3 fatty acid) and vitamins A and D, nutrients that improve the quality of tears and help them lubricate more effectively.

Also helpful: BioTears, an oral supplement that includes curcumin and other eye-protecting ingredients. (I am on the scientific advisory board of BioSyntrx, which makes BioTears and Eye & Body Complete, mentioned below, but I have no financial interest in the company.) I have found improvement in about 80% of patients who take BioTears. Follow the directions on the label.

Cataracts

Cataracts typically are caused by the age-related clumping of proteins in the crystalline lens of the eyes. More than half of Americans will have cataracts by the time they're 80.

What to do: Eat spinach, kale and other dark leafy greens every day. They contain lutein, an antioxidant that reduces the free-radical damage that increases cataract risk. (Lutein and zeaxanthin, another antioxidant, are the only carotenoids that concentrate in the lenses of the eyes.)

Important: Cook kale or other leafy greens with a little bit of oil…or eat them with a meal that contains olive oil or other fats. The carotenoids are fat-soluble, so they require a little fat for maximal absorption.

I also advise patients to take 500 milligrams (mg) of vitamin C three or four times a day (cut back if you get diarrhea). One study found that those who took vitamin C supplements for 10 years were 64% less likely to have cataracts.

The supplement Eye & Body Complete contains a mix of eye-protecting compounds, including bioflavonoids, bilberry and vitamins A and D. Follow instructions on the label.

Computer Vision Syndrome

The National Institute of Occupational Safety and Health reports that 88% of people who work at a computer for more than three hours a day complain of computer-related problems, including blurred vision, headaches, neck pain and eye dryness.

What to do: Take a supplement that contains about 6 mg of astaxanthin, a carotenoid. It reduces eyestrain by improving the stamina of eye muscles.

Also helpful: The 20/20/20 rule. After every 20 minutes on a computer, take 20 seconds and look 20 feet away.

Reduced Night Vision

True night blindness (nyctalopia) is rare in the US, but many older adults find that they struggle to see at night, which can make night driving difficult.

What to do: Take a daily supplement that includes one-half mg of copper and 25 mg of zinc. Zinc deficiencies have been associated with poor night vision—and you'll need the extra copper to "balance" the zinc. Zinc helps the body produce vitamin A, which is required by the retina to detect light.

Vitamin C and Cataract Risk

Vitamin C may reduce cataract risk. But the vitamin is most protective when it comes from food—not supplements.

Recent finding: Study participants with a higher dietary intake of vitamin C had one-third lower risk for cataracts than people who consumed the least vitamin C. Those who took vitamin C supplements showed no significant risk reduction.

Christopher Hammond, MD, Frost Chair of Ophthalmology at King's College London, UK, and leader of a study of 2,054 twins, published online in *Ophthalmology.*

Also helpful: The foods for AMD (below).

Age-Related Macular Degeneration (AMD)

This serious disease is the leading cause of blindness in older adults. Most people with AMD first will notice that their vision has become slightly hazy. As the disease progresses, it can cause a large blurred area in the center of the field of vision.

What to do: Eat several weekly servings of spinach or other brightly colored vegetables, such as kale and yellow peppers, or egg yolks. The nutrients and antioxidants in these foods can help slow the progression of AMD. The National Eye Institute's Age-Related Eye Disease Study (AREDS) reported that patients who already had macular degeneration and had adequate intakes of beta-carotene, zinc, copper and vitamins C and E were 25% less likely to develop an advanced form of the disease.

Also helpful: The Eye & Body Complete supplement, mentioned earlier. It contains all of the ingredients used in the original AREDS study—plus many others, including generous amounts of lutein and zeaxanthin that were included in a follow-up study, known as AREDS2—and was found to have positive effects.

Calendula for Cataracts

The late **James A. Duke, PhD,** an economic botanist retired from the USDA, where he developed a database on the health benefits of various plants (ARS-grin.gov/duke/). He is the author of numerous books including, most recently, *The Green Pharmacy Guide to Healing Foods: Proven Natural Remedies to Treat and Prevent More Than 80 Common Health Concerns.*

Calendula, or marigold, contains powerful plant-based carotenoids—particularly lutein and zeaxanthin—that help protect the eyes. In addition to being powerful antioxidants, these two compounds absorb damaging blue-light wavelengths from the sun. Increased intake of lutein and zeaxanthin has been associated with reduced risk for cataracts.

Best uses: Calendula makes an excellent addition to homemade vegetable soup. If you prefer to use calendula in supplement form, follow label instructions.

Spinach and Macular Degeneration

Michael T. Murray, ND, a licensed naturopathic physician based in Paradise Valley, Arizona. Dr. Murray has published more than 30 books, including *Bottom Line's Encyclopedia of Healing Foods*, with coauthor Joseph Pizzorno, ND. DoctorMurray.com

As the US population ages, there's been a dramatic increase in age-related macular degeneration, a leading cause of blindness. Could a few weekly servings of spinach make a difference? There's good evidence that it might.

How spinach helps: Spinach is exceptionally high in lutein, a plant pigment that concentrates in the eyes and deflects damaging light from sunshine. Studies have found that people who consumed 6 mg of lutein daily—the amount in about one-half cup of cooked spinach—were 43% less likely to develop macular degeneration. Research published in *JAMA Ophthalmology* shows that people who consume generous amounts of lutein are also less likely to develop cataracts than those who eat less.

Important: Whether you prefer your spinach raw or cooked, be sure to have it with a little bit of oil or fat—a drizzle of olive oil is plenty—or a small amount of some other fat such as chopped nuts or avocado. Lutein is a fat-soluble nutrient, which means it is absorbed more efficiently when it's consumed with a little fat.

CHAPTER 3

Superfoods That Fight Cancer

Seven Foods Proven to Fight Cancer

David Grotto, RD, LDN, a registered dietitian and former spokesperson for the American Dietetic Association. He is founder and president of Nutrition Housecall, LLC, a Chicago-area consulting firm specializing in family nutrition programs. He writes the "Ask the Guy-a-titian" column for *Chicago Wellness Magazine* and is author of *The Best Thing You Can Eat* and *101 Foods That Could Save Your Life*.

U p to one-third of all cancers could be prevented if people adopted healthier lifestyles, including eating healthier foods. *For even better odds, choose these seven specific foods that have been proven to prevent cancer...*

Cabbage

It's high in anticarcinogenic compounds called glucosinolates. Raw cabbage, particularly when it is fermented as sauerkraut, also is a good source of indole-3-carbinol (I3C), a substance that promotes the elimination of carcinogens from the body.

The Polish Women's Health Study, which looked at hundreds of Polish women in the US, found that those who had eaten four or more servings per week of raw, lightly cooked or fermented cabbage during adolescence were 72% less likely to develop breast cancer than women who had eaten only one-and-a-half servings per week. High consumption of cabbage during adulthood also provided significant protection even if little cabbage was eaten at a young age.

Recommended: Three or more one-half-cup servings per week of cabbage, cooked or raw.

Alternatives: Any cruciferous vegetable, including brussels sprouts, cauliflower, kale and broccoli. A recent study found that men who ate at least three servings per week of broccoli or other cruciferous vegetables were 41% less likely to get prostate cancer than men who ate less than one serving per week. Kimchi, a Korean pickled dish that is similar to sauerkraut, also is a good choice.

Flaxseeds

Little seeds with a nutty flavor, flaxseeds contain lignans, compounds that act like a weak form of estrogen. One study found that women with high levels of enterolactone (linked to a high intake of lignans) had a 58% lower risk for breast cancer. Flaxseeds also contain omega-3 fatty acids, which appear to inhibit colon cancer in both men and women.

Recommended: One to two tablespoons of ground flaxseed daily. You can sprinkle it on cereal or yogurt or add it to soups or stews.

Alternatives: Two or more servings per week of cold-water fish, such as mackerel or salmon, provide cancer-fighting amounts of omega-3s.

For more lignans: Eat walnuts, and cook with canola oil.

Mushrooms

The common white button mushroom found in supermarkets contains anticancer compounds. Scientists who compared vegetable extracts in the lab found that an extract made from white button mushrooms was the most effective at blocking aromatase, an enzyme that promotes breast cancer. Button mushrooms also appear to suppress the growth of prostate cancer cells.

Recommended: One-half cup of button mushrooms, three or four times per week.

Alternatives: Porcinis or chanterelles, wild mushrooms with a nuttier taste.

Olives

A Spanish laboratory study found that two compounds in olives—maslinic acid and oleanolic acid—inhibit the proliferation of cancer cells and promote apoptosis, the death of these cells. Other studies suggest that people who eat olives as part of a classic Mediterranean diet have lower rates of a variety of cancers, including colon cancer.

Recommended: Eight olives a day, green or black.

Alternative: One to two tablespoons of extra-virgin olive oil daily. Drizzle it on salad or vegetables to enhance absorption of their healthy nutrients.

Onions

When researchers compared the 10 vegetables most frequently consumed in the US, onions had the third-highest level of phenolic compounds, which are thought to be among the most potent anticancer substances found in foods.

In a Finnish study, men who frequently ate onions, apples and other foods high in quercetin (a phenolic compound) were 60% less likely to develop lung cancer than men who ate smaller amounts. Quercetin also appears to reduce the risk for liver and colon cancers.

Recommended: One-half cup of onions, cooked or raw, three times per week. Yellow and red onions contain the most cancer-preventing substances.

Alternatives: Apples, capers and green and black tea, all of which are high in quercetin. Garlic, a botanical relative of onions, provides many of the same active ingredients.

Pumpkin

Pumpkin, like all winter squash, is extremely high in carotenoids, including beta-carotene. A long-running Japanese study that looked at more than 57,000 participants found that people who ate the most pumpkin had lower rates of gastric, breast, lung and colorectal cancers. There also is some evidence that pumpkin seeds can help reduce the risk for prostate cancer.

Recommended: Three or more one-half-cup servings per week. Pumpkin can be baked like any winter squash.

Alternatives: Carrots, broccoli and all of the winter squashes, including acorn, butternut and spaghetti squash.

Raspberries

All of the foods that end with "erry"—including cherry, blueberry and straw-berry—contain anti-inflammatory compounds that reduce cell damage that can lead to cancer. Raspberries are higher in fiber than most berries and are an excellent source of ellagic acid and selenium, both of which protect against a variety of cancers.

Recent studies have shown that raspberries (or raspberry extract) inhibit both oral and liver cancer cells. The responses in these studies were dose-dependent—the more raspberry extract used, the greater the effect.

Recommended: One-and-a-half cups of raspberries, two or three times per week.

Alternative: Cherries (and cherry juice) contain about as much ellagic acid as raspberries. Frozen berries and cherries, which contain less water, provide a higher concentration of protective compounds than fresh ones.

Enjoy Your Chili—and Fight Cancer, Too!

Alice Bender, MS, RDN, head of Nutrition Programs for the American Institute for Cancer Research, a Washington, DC–based nonprofit devoted to research and education related to the role of nutrition in reducing cancer risk. Bender is also coauthor of the "Nutrition and Cancer Prevention" chapter in the reference book *Oncology Nutrition for Clinical Practice.*

Who doesn't love warming up after a cold winter day with a bowl of hot chili? With a seemingly endless list of potential ingredients—beans, meats, veggies, spices and even surprise additions such as chocolate or coffee—there's something for everyone.

A perk we shouldn't overlook: Even though chili is beloved mostly as a comfort food, the mainstay ingredients of many scrumptious chili recipes (such as beans, tomatoes, chili peppers and garlic) are packed with cancer-fighting properties. The recipes below are hearty enough to stand on their own...or you can round them out with a green salad packed with colorful veggies.

Curry Fights Skin Cancer

In a lab study of human cells, curcumin (the compound that makes curry yellow) was shown to interfere with the development of melanoma cells. Past studies have shown that people who eat curry in abundance have lower rates of lung, colon, prostate and breast cancers.

Theory: Curcumin curbs inflammation, a risk factor for cancer. Self-defense: Eat a half-tablespoon of curry daily.

Bharat B. Aggarwal, PhD, professor of cancer medicine, University of Texas M.D. Anderson Cancer Center, Houston.

LIME AND CHICKEN CHILI WITH AVOCADO

This Mexican-inspired chili gets a tart kick from limes, an excellent source of antioxidant vitamin C and anticancer phytochemicals such as limonoids and flavonoids. Tomatoes, beans and yellow corn add more cancer-protective fiber and phytonutrients. Garlic is rich in anticancer substances like quercetin and allicin.

Ingredients:

2 Tablespoons of extra-virgin olive oil

1 large chopped yellow onion

3 stalks of thinly sliced celery

1 seeded, diced jalapeño pepper

5 minced garlic cloves

1 pound of whole boneless, skinless chicken breasts

1 cup of frozen corn

1 14.5-ounce can of no-salt diced tomatoes

1 16-ounce can of cannellini beans (drained and rinsed)

4 cups of reduced-sodium chicken broth

1½ teaspoons of Italian seasoning

1 teaspoon of oregano

¼ teaspoon of cumin

2 whole limes

½ bunch of rinsed, chopped cilantro

1 medium avocado (cubed)

Directions: In a soup pot, heat the extra-virgin olive oil over medium-high heat. Sauté the onion, celery, jalapeño pepper and garlic cloves until tender—about six minutes. Then add the whole chicken breasts, corn, tomatoes, cannellini beans, chicken broth, Italian seasoning, oregano and cumin to the pot. Stir the ingredients. Bring to a boil, then reduce heat, cover and simmer for 55 minutes. Transfer the chicken breasts to a large platter, shred them with two forks and return the chicken meat to the pot. Before serving, stir in the juice from one of the limes and the cilantro. Ladle the chili into bowls and garnish each serving with cubed avocado and a wedge from the remaining lime. Makes six savory servings.

SWEET POTATO CHILI WITH PEANUTS

This bean-free chili is a good option for people who find that beans make them gassy. Sweet potatoes are a true superfood, brimming with plant pigments that have been shown in lab studies to help prevent abnormal cell growth and the

---

The Healthy Plate Formula to Fight Cancer

To help fight cancer, it's important to make wise food choices throughout the day.

Here's how: Fill half your plate with vegetables (organic, if possible) at every meal, including breakfast. The other half should contain protein, fruits (preferably organic) and whole grains. Try replacing meat with sardines, salmon and other cold-water fish (loaded with omega-3 fatty acids) and beans at least four times a week for a healthy source of animal and plant proteins. Add spices and herbs, which are filled with healthy phytochemicals. It's also smart to eat fewer "white" foods, including white bread, white rice, etc. These and other high-glycemic foods are quickly converted to glucose, which increases levels of insulin and insulin-like growth factor (a cancer promoter).

Helpful: Meet with a dietitian to help guide you in healthy eating. To find a registered dietitian near you, consult the Academy of Nutrition and Dietetics, EatRight.org.

Lorenzo Cohen, PhD, the Richard E. Haynes Distinguished Professor in Clinical Cancer Prevention and director of the Integrative Medicine Program at The University of Texas MD Anderson Cancer Center in Houston.

formation of cancer-promoting free radicals. Peanuts add a hearty flavor while providing some protein and fiber.

Ingredients:

½ medium chopped yellow onion

1 thinly sliced, peeled carrot

½ seeded, chopped green bell pepper

½ seeded, chopped red bell pepper

1 Tablespoon of canola oil

1–2 minced garlic cloves

2 pounds of sweet potatoes (peeled or unpeeled and cut into bite-size chunks—about 2 cups)

¾ cup of unsalted roasted peanuts

1 14.5-ounce can of no-salt crushed tomatoes

½ 6-ounce can of tomato paste

1 4-ounce can of diced mild green chili peppers

2–3 Tablespoons of chili powder

½ Tablespoon of cumin

½ Tablespoon of sugar

Optional: For extra flavor and an antioxidant boost, add one tablespoon of unsweetened cocoa powder or one-half cup of strong brewed coffee.

Directions: In a large, heavy pot, sauté the onion, carrot, and green and red bell peppers in canola oil over medium heat until the onion is golden—about eight minutes. Add the garlic cloves and stir constantly for 30 seconds. Stir in the chunked sweet potatoes, peanuts, crushed tomatoes (and juice), tomato paste and green chili peppers (with liquid). Next, add the chili powder, cumin and sugar. Add water as needed. Bring the mixture to a boil, then reduce the heat to low and simmer gently, stirring occasionally, for 15 to 25 minutes, until the potatoes are tender. Season to taste with salt and pepper. Makes five mouthwatering servings.

Red Chili Pepper Fights Cancer

Sanjay K. Srivastava, PhD, associate professor of biomedical sciences Texas Tech University Health Sciences Center School of Pharmacy, Amarillo, Texas.

It contains capsaicin, an anti-inflammatory that is effective against cancer cells. In tests, capsaicin caused cancer cells to die without damaging normal ones. Though clinical trials are needed before a recommendation to eat chili pepper can be made, it can be enjoyed as part of your regular diet.

Magical Miso: 10 Ways to Cook with an Umami Powerhouse

Debby Maugans, food writer based in Asheville, North Carolina, and author of *Small Batch Baking, Small Batch Baking for Chocolate Lovers* and *Farmer and Chef Asheville.*

Miso, the traditional Japanese fermented soybean paste we know best in miso soup, is intensely flavorful, nutritious, cancer-protective, packed with good-for-you probiotics—and remarkably versatile in the kitchen.

Here's what you need to know to maximize both health benefits and flavor with this ancient superfood—10 recipe inspirations, including a quick-and-easy everyday vegetable soup.

Maximizing Miso

Both the culinary and the health benefits of miso stem from the fermentation process. To make miso, steamed soybeans and grains (such as rice and barley), along with salt, is inoculated with a fungi known as koji (Aspergillus oryzae) and allowed to ferment over several months—like wine or beer.

Koji fermentation allows beneficial bacteria (probiotics) to develop and also breaks down the cancer-protective isoflavones in soy to make them easier for our bodies to use.

Fermentation also intensifies the flavor. Miso is rich in umami—the "fifth" taste that adds depth to foods. Foods high on the umami scale, such as aged Parmesan cheese and roasted meats, taste rich, earthy and complex. It's a subtle flavor that blends well with others, expanding and rounding them out. Umami flavors are literally mouthwatering—they stimulate saliva, which enhances appetite and digestion.

A few tips to make the best use of miso for flavor and health...

•**Look for miso that is produced by the traditional, artisanal method.** Check labels, and avoid any that contain MSG. Some products use fermentation accelerants, but you'll get more probiotics when your miso is aged naturally. Look for it in natural foods stores and natural-food–oriented supermarkets.

•**The longer the fermentation, the more probiotics.** Products aged 180 days or more have the most probiotics. This is a darker (often red), richer, earthy and savory miso. It's great in wintry foods such as hearty soups and roasted meats.

•**Lighter miso, often white or yellow, has its place, too.** It has a sweeter, more subtle flavor. Use it in vinaigrettes and with grilled chicken and vegetables. It's good to use in the summer.

•**Miso is high is salt, so use it sparingly.** One or two teaspoons per serving will enhance a food's flavor without overpowering it.

•**You can warm miso paste, but don't simmer it—and definitely don't boil it.** That kills the probiotics. It's best to add it to dishes at the end of the cooking process—after the pot has been removed from the heat.

Ten Ways to Cook with Miso

You'll be amazed at the layers of flavor miso builds in the following recipe ideas...

1. Miso Pesto. Combine in a blender or food processor 1 cup packed basil leaves, 2–4 cloves garlic, ¼ cup toasted walnuts, ¼ cup packed parsley leaves, 2 tablespoons white miso and ¼ cup extra-virgin olive oil. Pulse, leaving some texture. Serve with cooked shrimp, cooked pasta, grilled chicken.

2. Sriracha Miso BBQ Sauce. Whisk together 5 Tablespoons packed brown sugar, ¼ cup Sriracha sauce, 3 Tablespoons miso, 2 Tablespoons sesame oil and 2 Tablespoons rice wine vinegar. Serve with grilled tofu or chicken.

3. Thai Miso Peanut Sauce. Combine in a small saucepan ¼ cup miso, 3 Tablespoons peanut butter, 2 Tablespoons fresh lemon juice, ⅓ cup water, 1 Tablespoon dry sherry (optional), 2 teaspoons grated fresh ginger and ½ teaspoon spicy sesame oil. Cook and stir over medium heat until hot. Serve with soba noodles, kebabs or grilled chicken.

4. Miso Maple "Caramel" Sauce. Heat ½ cup maple syrup and 1 Tablespoon white miso in a small saucepan (don't simmer or boil it). Serve over ice cream or pancakes.

5. Red Miso Chickpea Hummus. Process in a food processor until smooth: 1 cup cooked chickpeas, ¼ cup diced roasted red bell pepper or pimiento, 2 Tablespoons white miso, 2 Tablespoons tahini, 1½ Tablespoons fresh lemon juice and 2 cloves minced garlic. Serve as a dip or sandwich spread.

6. Miso Sesame Salad Dressing. Whisk together 1½ tablespoons white miso, 2 Tablespoons rice vinegar, 1½ Tablespoons fresh orange juice, 1 Tablespoon dark sesame oil and 2 teaspoons grated fresh ginger. Cover and chill. Serve with greens or drizzle on grilled chicken or fish.

7. Miso Balsamic Glazed Roasted Vegetables. Mix 2 Tablespoons red or white miso, 1 Tablespoon balsamic vinegar, 1 Tablespoon water and 2 teaspoons olive oil. Brush on cut vegetables before roasting.

8. Better Miso Burger. Mix 2 Tablespoons red or white miso with 2 Tablespoons water and mix into 1 pound of ground beef, lamb or turkey. Form into burgers and grill.

9. Raspberry Miso Sauce. Thaw 1 cup of frozen raspberries in a small saucepan. Add 2 teaspoons honey, and cook over low heat 5 minutes. Press through sieve over a bowl. Stir 2 teaspoons miso and 1 teaspoon balsamic vinegar into the juice. Spoon over fish fillets after cooking or baste shrimp after grilling. Also delicious over frozen yogurt.

10. Vegetable Miso Soup. Miso adds a slight sweetness and depth of flavor to this broth-based soup. For a variation, serve with a squeeze of lime and a sprinkling of cilantro leaves. You can also add cubed firm tofu along with the carrots to make it a protein-rich main dish.

Makes 9 cups, or 4 to 5 servings

¼ cup miso

5 cups plus 2 Tablespoons low-sodium vegetable broth, divided

1 Tablespoon grated fresh ginger

2 teaspoons grated fresh garlic

¾ cup sliced carrots

1 cup very thinly sliced cremini mushrooms

1½ cups packed chopped fresh kale

1 cup very thinly sliced Brussels sprouts

1 cup hot, cooked soba noodles

Stir together miso and 2 Tablespoons of the broth in a small bowl.

Combine remaining 5 cups of the broth, ginger and garlic in a medium saucepan. Bring to a boil, cover and reduce heat—simmer for one minute. Add carrots, cover and simmer for three minutes. Add mushrooms, cover and cook until the carrots are tender—4 to 5 minutes. Add kale and Brussels sprouts, cover and cook briefly to wilt and blanch them—about one minute.

Remove saucepan from heat, and stir in miso mixture and soba noodles. Serve immediately.

Magical Food Combos That Fight Cancer

Karen Collins, RD, registered dietitian and nutrition adviser to the American Institute for Cancer Research (AICR.org). A syndicated newspaper columnist and public speaker, she maintains a private nutrition counseling practice in Washington, DC.

Researchers know that some foods can help prevent cancer. Now there is growing evidence that certain food combinations may offer more protection against cancer than any one specific food.

The following combinations of foods are especially beneficial. *Eat them regularly—either at the same meal or separately throughout the week...*

Tomatoes and Broccoli

Results of an animal study presented at the American Institute for Cancer Research International Research Conference showed that rats with tumors that were given a diet of tomatoes and broccoli had significantly smaller tumors than animals fed one of these foods.

The lycopene in tomatoes is an antioxidant. Antioxidants are crucial for preventing cancer because they help prevent unstable molecules, called free radicals, from damaging cell structures and DNA. Broccoli contains chemical compounds known as glucosinolates, which may be effective in flushing carcinogens from the body.

Also helpful: Combine broccoli or other cruciferous vegetables, such as brussels sprouts and cabbage, with foods that are high in selenium, such as shellfish and Brazil nuts. A study published by the UK's Institute of Food Research found that the combination of broccoli's glucosinolates and selenium has more powerful anticancer effects than either food eaten alone.

Brussels Sprouts and Broccoli

These potent cancer-fighting vegetables also are rich in vitamin C and folate, as well as phytonutrients that deactivate carcinogens. When eaten in combination, brussels sprouts and broccoli may provide more protection than either one eaten alone.

Brussels sprouts have the phytonutrient *crambene*, which stimulates phase-2 enzymes, substances that help prevent carcinogens from damaging DNA. Broccoli is high in indole-3-carbinol, a phytonutrient that also stimulates phase-2 enzymes—but in a different way.

Oranges, Apples, Grapes and Blueberries

Each of these foods is very high in antioxidants. In a recent laboratory analysis, researchers measured the amount of antioxidants in each of these fruits individually. Then they combined them and took additional measurements.

Result: The mixture of fruits was more powerful against free radicals than any one fruit alone.

Curcumin and Quercetin

Curcumin is a phytonutrient found in the spice turmeric. Quercetin is a phytonutrient that is abundant in yellow onions, especially in the outermost rings. According to a small study in *Clinical Gastroenterology and Hepatology*, people who consumed large amounts of these two phytonutrients had a reduction in the number of colon polyps, growths that may turn into cancer.

The study looked at a small number of people with familial adenomatous polyposis, a hereditary condition that increases the likelihood of developing polyps. The phytochemical combination reduced the number of polyps by 60%. It also caused some polyps to shrink.

The researchers used concentrated forms of curcumin and quercetin. You would have to eat two-and-a-half tablespoons of turmeric daily to get a comparable amount. To get the necessary amount of quercetin, you would need to have about two-thirds cup of chopped onions daily.

Recommended: Eat a variety of herbs and spices to get the most phytonutrient protection. Even small amounts used frequently will impact your health over time. Among herbs, rosemary and oregano rank among the best phytonutrient sources. Ginger is another powerful spice.

Tomatoes and Fat

The lycopene in tomatoes is particularly effective against prostate cancer, but only when it's consumed with a small amount of fat. Lycopene, like other members of the carotenoid chemical family, is a fat-soluble substance. The body can't absorb it efficiently in the absence of fat.

It takes only three to five grams of fat (about one teaspoon of oil) to improve the absorption of lycopene from tomatoes. For example, you could have a salad with an oil-based dressing. The type of fat doesn't matter for absorption of lycopene and other carotenoids, but you might as well choose a fat that promotes health. Olive oil and canola oil are good choices.

More Variety, Less Cancer

In a study published in *The Journal of Nutrition*, researchers divided 106 women into two groups. All of the women were asked to eat eight to 10 servings of fruits and vegetables daily for two weeks. However, one of the groups (the high-diversity group) was told to include foods from 18 different botanical groups, including onions and garlic from the allium family, legumes, cruciferous vegetables, etc. The other group (the low-diversity one) was asked to concentrate all its choices among only five major groups.

Beer Marinade Helps Reduce Cancer Risk

A beer marinade makes grilled meat healthier.

Recent finding: Marinating meat in beer before grilling reduces polycyclic aromatic hydrocarbons (PAHs), the cancer-causing carcinogens that are created when meat is cooked on a grill.

Best: After a four-hour marinade, dark beer reduced PAHs by 53%. Nonalcoholic pilsner reduced PAHs by 25%, while alcoholic pilsner reduced PAHs by only 13% compared with grilling with no beer.

Study by researchers at University of Porto, Portugal, published in *Journal of Agricultural and Food Chemistry.*

Results: Women in both groups showed a decrease in lipid peroxidation—important for reducing the risk of cancer and heart disease. However, only the women in the high-diversity group showed a decrease in DNA oxidation, one of the steps that initiates cancer development.

The ways that chemicals work in the body, known as metabolic pathways, have a rate-limiting effect. This means that beyond a certain point, eating more of a specific food won't provide additional protection. Eating a wide variety of foods brings more metabolic pathways into play, thus bypassing this limiting effect.

Cancer-Fighting Superfoods: What to Eat Before, During and After Chemotherapy

Rebecca Katz, MS, senior chef-in-residence and nutrition educator at Commonweal Cancer Help Program in Bolinas, California. She is founder of Inner Cook, a Bay Area culinary practice that works with cancer patients, and executive chef for The Center for Mind-Body Medicine's Food as Medicine and CancerGuides Professional Training Programs. She is author, with Mat Edelson, of *The Cancer-Fighting Kitchen: Nourishing, Big-Flavor Recipes for Cancer Treatment and Recovery.* RebeccaKatz.com

Some people experience virtually no side effects from cancer chemotherapy, but this is rare. Most patients report at least some problems, including nausea, fatigue and diarrhea during the treatment.

Reason: The drugs that are used in chemotherapy are designed to kill fast-growing cancer cells. But they also damage fast-growing healthy cells, particularly in the mouth, digestive tract and hair follicles.

Good nutrition is critical if you're undergoing chemotherapy. It's estimated that up to 80% of cancer patients are malnourished. People who eat well before and during chemotherapy tend to have fewer side effects. They also are more likely to complete the full course of therapy than those who are poorly nourished and may feel too sick to continue. *What to do…*

•**Load up on nutrient-rich foods.** In the weeks before chemotherapy, patients should emphasize nutrient-dense foods, such as whole grains, vegetables and legumes. The high nutrient load of a healthy diet helps strengthen healthy cells so that they're better able to withstand—and then recover from—the effects of chemotherapy. Good choices…

•**Dark leafy greens,** such as spinach, kale and Swiss chard. They're high in antioxidants, such as beta-carotene, lutein and other phytonutrients. These compounds help minimize the damaging effects of free radicals, tissue-damaging molecules that are produced in large amounts during chemotherapy. Kale is particularly good because it contains indole-3-carbinol, a compound that has anticancer properties.

•**Olive oil,** like green vegetables, is high in antioxidants. It's one of the best sources of oleic acid, an omega-9 fatty acid that strengthens cell membranes and improves the ability of the immune system to fight cancer cells. I like extra-virgin olive oil because it has been exposed to the least heat.

•**Garlic.** The National Cancer Institute reports that people who eat garlic regularly seem to have a lower risk for intestinal and other cancers, including breast cancer. The strong-tasting sulfur compounds in garlic, such as allicin, have strong antiviral and antibacterial effects—important for chemotherapy patients because they're susceptible to infection. In my recipes, I use fresh garlic. I smash it and let it sit for 10 minutes to allow the antiviral properties to become more accessible—then chop and cook. (To smash garlic, set the side of a chef's knife on the clove, place the heel of your hand on the flat side of the knife and apply pressure.)

•**Increase protein.** It's the main structural component of muscle and other tissues. People who undergo chemotherapy need large amounts of protein to repair tissue damage that occurs during the treatments.

Recommended: About 80 grams of protein daily. That's nearly double the amount that healthy adults need. Cancer patients who increase their protein about a week before chemotherapy, and continue to get extra protein afterward, recover more quickly. They also will have more energy and less fatigue.

Try this: Two or more daily smoothies (made in a blender with juice or milk, a variety of fresh fruits and ice, if you like) that are supplemented with a scoop of whey protein powder. The protein in whey is easily absorbed by the intestine. And most people can enjoy a nutrient-rich smoothie even when they have nausea or digestive problems related to chemotherapy.

•**Drink to reduce discomfort.** Stay hydrated both before and after chemotherapy sessions to reduce nausea. Drink liquids until your urine runs clear—if it has more than a hint of yellow, you need to drink more.

Helpful: Soups and broths provide water, as well as protein, minerals and vitamins.

•**Avoid your favorite foods two days before treatments.** It's common for chemotherapy patients to develop food aversions when they get nauseated from treatments and then to associate the nausea with certain foods. It's sad when people develop aversions and can never again enjoy their favorite foods.

•**Eat lightly and frequently.** People tend to experience more nausea when the stomach is empty. During and after "chemo days," keep something in your stomach all the time—but not too much. Patients do better when they have a light snack, such as sautéed vegetables or a bowl of broth, than when they go hungry or eat a lot at one sitting.

•**Treat with ginger.** When your stomach is upset, steep three slices of fresh ginger in a cup of simmering water for 10 minutes, then drink the tea. Or grate fresh ginger with a very fine grater, such as a Microplane, and put the shavings under your tongue. Ginger alleviates nausea almost instantly.

●**Overcome "metal mouth."** The drugs used in chemotherapy can damage the nerves that control the taste buds. Some people complain about a metallic taste in their mouths after treatments. Others notice that foods taste "flat" or that their mouths are extremely sensitive to hot or cold.

These changes, known as transient taste changes, usually disappear a few weeks (or, in some cases, months) after treatments, but they can make it difficult for people to eat in the meantime.

Helpful: The FASS method. It stands for Fat, Acid, Salt and Sweet. Most people will find that it's easier to enjoy their meals, and therefore ingest enough nutrients, when they combine one or more of these elements in every meal.

For fat, add more olive oil than usual to meals…lemons are a good source of acid…sea salt has less of a chemical aftertaste than regular salt…and maple syrup gives sweetness with more nutrients (including immune-building manganese and zinc) than table sugar.

●**Try kudzu root.** Used in a powder form to thicken sauces, puddings and other foods, it soothes the intestine and can help prevent diarrhea. You also can dissolve one teaspoon of kudzu root in one teaspoon of cold liquid and drink that. Drink after meals, as needed. Kudzu root is available in most health-food stores.

●**Soothe mouth sores** with soft, easy-to-eat foods, such as granitas (similar to "Italian ices") or smoothies. The sores can be intensely painful, which makes it difficult to eat.

Recommended: Watermelon ice cubes. Purée watermelon, and put it in a tray to freeze. Then suck on the cubes. The cold acts like a topical anesthetic—you can numb the mouth before eating a regular meal. And the juice from the melon is just as hydrating as water but provides extra nutrients, including the antioxidant lycopene.

Beat Cancer with This Bean

David Grotto, RD, LDN, a registered dietitian and founder and president of Nutrition Housecall, LLC, a Chicago-based nutrition consulting firm that provides nutrition communications, lecturing and consulting services, along with personalized, at-home dietary services. He is author of *The Best Things You Can Eat*. DavidGrotto.com

Many people think of broccoli and other cruciferous vegetables as the best cancer-fighting foods. These are excellent choices…but they are not the best.

**Foods That Help Prevent
Lung Cancer**

Apples, tomatoes and oranges provide antioxidants that help nourish the lungs. Carrots, yellow squash and dark, leafy greens provide antioxidants called carotenoids that protect lung tissue. Water helps flush out toxins. Whole-soy foods contain phytoestrogens that may have a protective effect.

Still the number-one recommendation: Do not smoke.

DrWeil.com

Best food: Black beans. They're high in anthocyanins and triterpenoids, potent antioxidants that can reduce cell-damaging inflammation and possibly increase the destruction of abnormal cells.

All beans with vivid colors—such as kidney beans (red), pinto beans (brown) and adzuki beans (deep red)—contain these cancer-fighting compounds.

What to do: Eat at least three cups of cooked beans a week. One study found that people who ate beans more than twice a week were 47% less likely to develop colon cancer than those who ate them less than once a week.

Also helpful: Tomatoes in all forms, including ketchup and tomato paste. Tomatoes are rich in lycopene, a compound that appears to reduce the risk for prostate cancer. Cooked tomatoes actually provide more lycopene than fresh. But don't overdo ketchup—it's loaded with sugar and salt.

Arugula Fights Cancer

Michael T. Murray, ND, a licensed naturopathic physician based in Paradise Valley, Arizona. Dr. Murray has published more than 30 books, including *Bottom Line's Encyclopedia of Healing Foods,* with coauthor Joseph Pizzorno, ND. DoctorMurray.com

Arugula is a peppery green with a sharp taste that adds a distinctive zip to otherwise bland salads. The pungent flavor has earned it the nickname "salad rocket."

The zesty flavor of arugula is largely due to its high concentration of sulfur-containing compounds. We think of arugula as a salad green, but it's actually a crucifer—in the same plant family as superfoods such as broccoli, cabbage and kale. Like other crucifers, it contains a group of anticancer compounds known as glucosinolates, which have detoxifying effects.

How arugula helps: Compounds in arugula, including sulforaphane and indole-3-carbinol, increase the body's excretion of a form of estrogen that has been linked to breast cancer. A Chinese study found that women who regularly ate a daily serving of cruciferous vegetables were 50% less likely to develop breast cancer. Another study found that just one weekly serving was enough to reduce cancer risk (including oral, colorectal and kidney malignancies).

Bonus: The sulforaphane in arugula has another benefit. It appears to help the body eliminate H. pylori, a bacterium that causes most peptic ulcers and greatly increases the risk for gastric cancer.

Foods That Fight Colon Cancer

Jung Han Yoon Park, PhD, professor in the department of food, science and nutrition at Hallym University in Chuncheon, South Korea.

Have you ever heard of a nutrient called luteolin? It's one of the lesser-known flavonoids, chemical compounds that are found in many vegetables and herbs, and a recent study showed luteolin's ability to stop colon cancer cells in their tracks. This is potentially big news.

Stopping Cancer in Its Tracks

Colon cancer cells—unlike many other cancer cells—are continually exposed to the foods we eat. Previous studies showed that luteolin could cause colon cancer cells to die, but no one knew how it did that, or if luteolin could also cause normal, healthy intestinal cells to die in the process.

Researchers conducted a petri dish study and created three groups. One group contained human colon cancer cells and luteolin...the second group contained human colon cancer cells alone...and the third group contained noncancerous intestinal epithelial cells from rats (because it's difficult to culture healthy human intestinal cells) and luteolin.

The researchers were looking to see whether luteolin affected cancerous and noncancerous cells—and more importantly, how. The results were clear after only one day. By counting the number of cells in the dishes, the researchers found that, as expected, human colon cancer cells that were exposed to luteolin stopped multiplying, while human cancer cells that were not exposed to luteolin kept multiplying. And noncancerous intestinal epithelial cells from rats were not adversely affected by luteolin, which was great news.

So how did plain old luteolin—remember, it's just a natural part of vegetables—have such a large impact on the human colon cancer cells? With more analysis, the researchers discovered that luteolin interfered with an insulin-like growth factor (IGF). Next, researchers are expected to test the effect of luteolin on live animals with colon cancer, probably mice. If that goes well, human tests will quickly follow.

Eat It Up

But there's no need to wait for further studies to be done to eat foods containing luteolin—especially if you have colon cancer or are at high risk for it. You're probably eating at least a little bit of it already, and there's no harm in eating more by increasing your intake of certain foods and herbs. Parsley and thyme are unusually rich in luteolin (containing more than 50 milligrams per 100 grams). Foods that have 10 to 50 milligrams per 100 grams include peppermint leaves and rutabagas. And others that have small amounts of luteolin include chives, artichokes, broccoli, carrots, peppers (both hot and sweet), beets, Brussels sprouts, cabbage, cauliflower, lettuce, apple skins, basil, chamomile tea and spinach.

Taking a luteolin supplement right now isn't recommended because more studies need to be done to establish a safe dosage.

Researchers don't yet know how much luteolin-rich food one would have to eat for it to be beneficial, but don't be shy about it—fill up your plate because you aren't going to get too much luteolin from food. Because luteolin isn't affected by heat, it doesn't matter whether you eat the vegetables raw or cooked. So serve them up any way you like!

CHAPTER 4

Superfoods to Fight Allergies and Respiratory Conditions

The Superfoods That Relieve Allergies to Pollen, Dust, Mold

Leo Galland, MD, director of the Foundation for Integrated Medicine in New York City. He has held faculty positions at Rockefeller University, Albert Einstein College of Medicine and State University of New York, Stony Brook. He is coauthor of *The Allergy Solution: Unlock the Surprising, Hidden Truth About Why You Are Sick* and *How to Get Well.* DrGalland.com

The right foods can help relieve allergies to dust, pollen, mold and other spores in the air—easing symptoms that include sneezing, stuffy nose and wheezing.

Recent finding: Allergy symptoms are less common on the rural Greek island of Crete than elsewhere in Greece, even though there's no shortage of allergens blowing around. According to a study published in *Thorax*, the people of Crete can thank their diet. Researchers tested 690 island children for airborne allergies and asked their parents to answer questions about their children's diets and symptoms. Eighty percent of the children ate fruit at least twice a day, and 68% ate vegetables that often. Those who ate more nuts, grapes, oranges, apples and tomatoes—the main local products—had fewer allergy symptoms than those who ate less.

Allergy symptoms occur when an overactive immune system responds to harmless substances as if they could cause disease. Inflammation is an early step in the immune response. Most of the foods that relieve allergies are anti-inflammatory, modulating the immune system response.

Foods That Fight Allergies

The following foods help battle airborne allergies...

•**Fruits high in vitamin C, an antioxidant, may help reduce inflammation.** Year-round, eat two pieces of fruit daily. When you're especially congested, choose from these twice a day—an orange, one cup of strawberries, an apple, one cup of grapes or a medium-sized wedge of watermelon. Bonus: The skins of red grapes are loaded with the antioxidant resveratrol and were found to relieve wheezing in the Crete study.

•**Nuts, especially almonds, hazelnuts and peanuts, are a good source of vitamin E, which helps minimize inflammation.** Eat a single one-ounce serving of any of these nuts daily year-round to help prevent symptoms. If you do have symptoms, increase the servings—try two tablespoons of peanut butter and one ounce each of hazelnuts and almonds a day.

•**Cold-water fish (wild salmon, mackerel, trout, herring and sardines), as well as walnuts and flaxseed, contain omega-3 fatty acids, which help fight inflammation.** Eat at least two servings of cold-water fish each week year-round and three servings during the seasons when you experience airborne allergies. Also have 12 walnuts and one tablespoon of ground flaxseed a day.

•**Oysters, shrimp and crab,** as well as legumes, whole grains and tofu, are all high in zinc, which has antibacterial and antiviral effects that provide relief for immune systems overtaxed by fighting allergies. Have six oysters, six shrimp or a few crabs every week, and twice that when your allergies bother you. Also have one serving of whole grains and one of beans or tofu a day.

•**Tea, whether green, white or black, is full of flavonoids, plant compounds that reduce inflammation.** Tea also increases proteins in the body that fight infection, again relieving an overtaxed immune system. Enjoy one cup daily, and increase to two when your allergies are a problem.

Helpful: Drink your tea first thing in the morning with lemon and honey to stimulate the cilia—the tiny hairs in the nose that sweep pollen and dust out of the way.

•**Horseradish, hot mustard, fennel, anise and sage also stimulate the cilia and act as natural decongestants.** Add a dash to food whenever possible.

Foods to Avoid All Year

If you experience congestion or other symptoms year-round, ask an allergist to conduct a skin test to identify allergies to dust, mold and foods. *Then consider the following changes in your daily diet...*

●**Mold and yeast in food can aggravate an allergy to mold in the air.** If you're allergic to mold, avoid foods that contain yeast, such as bread and baked goods (unless they are labeled "yeast free")…wine, beer and spirits…fermented foods, such as sauerkraut and cider…foods that tend to get moldy, such as cheese and mushrooms…vinegar and sauces that contain vinegar, such as mayonnaise, barbecue sauce, mustard and salad dressing.

Helpful: Use lemon juice and spices in dressings instead.

●**Milk and dairy products,** such as yogurt, butter and ice cream, could be making you feel worse if you have a congested nose year-round, a symptom typically caused by an allergy to dust. One explanation is that casein, the protein in milk, can promote the formation of mucus. Although there isn't strong science showing that milk aggravates congestion, it's worth experimenting by cutting dairy from your diet for at least two weeks. If your allergies improve when you avoid dairy products, eliminate dairy year-round. You will then need to take a calcium supplement, usually 1,000 milligrams (mg) a day, to compensate for the decreased calcium intake that accompanies a dairy-free diet.

●**Soy, corn and wheat.** Soy, including soy milk, tofu, soybean oil, edamame and soy sauce, may aggravate chronic congestion, according to clinical observation. Even if you don't appear allergic to soy on a skin-prick test, experiment by eliminating soy from your diet for at least two weeks.

The same is true of corn (including cornflakes, corn chips and corn oil) and wheat (including all breads and baked goods unless they are marked "wheat-free" or "gluten-free"). If you find that your symptoms are alleviated when you stop eating any of these foods, eliminate them year-round.

Papaya for Allergies

Mao Shing Ni, LaC, DOM, PhD, a Santa Monica, California–based licensed acupuncturist and doctor of oriental medicine. He is cofounder of Yo San University, an accredited graduate school of Traditional Chinese Medicine in Los Angeles, and author of *Secrets of Longevity.* TaoOfWellness.com

Papaya is rich in the enzyme bromelain and has long been used by the Chinese to help reduce the inflammatory process that promotes allergic reactions. Other bromelain-rich foods include pineapple and kiwifruit.

The Allergy-Fighting Diet

Leo Galland, MD, director of the Foundation for Integrated Medicine in New York City. He has held faculty positions at Rockefeller University, Albert Einstein College of Medicine and State University of New York, Stony Brook. He is coauthor of *The Allergy Solution: Unlock the Surprising, Hidden Truth About Why You Are Sick* and *How to Get Well.* DrGalland.com

The right diet can help relieve your allergies whether you're allergic to pollen, dust, mold, certain foods or other allergens. And it can relieve symptoms that you might not even know come from allergies—including fatigue, weight gain and depression. The key is to use foods to improve your immune response. *Here's how…*

Boost Your T-regs

Immune cells known as regulatory T-cells, or T-regs, limit inflammation and dampen the allergic response. The cells don't function properly in people with allergies, which can lead to a host of allergic symptoms.

If you know you're allergic to something, avoidance is an obvious solution. But many people don't know what they're allergic to—or even if they are allergic. You can use dietary changes to increase T-regs and dampen any allergic response.

Step 1: Three-Day Power Wash

I advise patients to completely give up the foods that commonly aggravate allergies. These include dairy (including yogurt), wheat, seafood, eggs, soy, nuts, peanuts, yeast (found in bread, alcohol, vinegar, commercial fruit juice and commercial soups and sauces) and nightshade vegetables (such as tomatoes, bell peppers, potatoes and eggplant).

This is not meant to be a permanent diet. You have to give up these foods for three days (unless you discover that you're allergic to a particular food, in which case you'll give it up altogether). Taking a break from likely offenders resets the immune system—it clears your body of potential allergens and lets you start with a clean slate.

For three days, you'll consume only the soup and the smoothie (see next page) that I developed for blunting the immune response (you'll also drink oolong tea). Have the smoothie for breakfast and a midafternoon snack. The soup is lunch and dinner. Eat until you are satisfied but not too full. Have your doctor look at the recipes to make sure that they are appropriate for you.

●**Immune balance smoothie.** In a blender, combine one cup of strawberries, one medium avocado, one cup of chopped arugula, one-half head of chopped romaine lettuce, two tablespoons of ground chia seeds and one cup of brewed green tea. If desired, add one medium banana.

Blend until smooth. The smoothie will become thicker and creamier if you refrigerate it after blending.

If you happen to be allergic to any of the ingredients, just leave it out.

●**Immune balance soup.** Sauté three cups of sliced carrots in three tablespoons of extra-virgin olive oil for 10 minutes. Add one cup of chopped parsley, two cups of chopped scallions (green parts only), 12 ounces of chopped broccoli, three ounces of chopped baby kale, one teaspoon of turmeric powder and one-quarter teaspoon of ground black pepper. Add salt to taste. Cook and stir for one minute. Add 12 cups of water, and bring to a boil. Cover and simmer for 20 minutes.

Add one tablespoon of shredded daikon radish just before serving.

●**Organic oolong tea.** I emphasize this tea for a specific reason. It's very high in catechins, which are flavonoids that inhibit allergic reactions—they're even stronger than the compounds in green tea. One study found that a majority of patients with allergic eczema who didn't respond to medications had significant improvements after drinking oolong tea for one to two weeks. Drink four cups daily (no more) during the Power Wash and a cup or two daily after that.

Step 2: Reintroduction

After three days, continue to enjoy the homemade smoothie and soup and organic oolong tea as you gradually reintroduce foods from your regular diet—a new food or food group each day. Start with foods that are less likely to provoke allergic reactions such as rice or free-range poultry, and gradually move toward the more allergenic foods such as nuts, seafood, eggs and dairy products, one group at a time. Keep notes about what you're eating and symptoms (if any) that you experience—including symptoms you don't typically associate with allergies (see page 71). This will help you determine whether particular foods—or ingredients in packaged foods—are triggering symptoms.

I've found that patients who give up problem foods for at least six months can sometimes eat them again, in small amounts, without having symptoms return. This doesn't apply to things such as sodas, candies or other junk foods, including commercially prepared pastries. These foods always contribute to allergies (including common dust and pollen allergies) by increasing inflammation and should be avoided.

Important: Consult your doctor before reintroducing foods, especially if you suffer from anaphylaxis or asthma or if you previously have experienced an adverse reaction to any of the foods.

Step 3: Immune Balance

No matter what you're allergic to, make an effort to eat healthier foods that fortify T-regs. *Most important…*

•**Natural folate.** Many foods are fortified with folic acid, an important (but synthetic) B vitamin. Natural sources of folate are better for T-reg function.

Examples: Leafy vegetables, legumes, peas, asparagus, cauliflower and brussels sprouts.

•**More flavonoids.** I believe that many of the inflammatory disorders that plague Americans, including allergies and asthma, are due in part to flavonoid deficiencies. Flavonoids, an important family of plant compounds, have anti-inflammatory and antioxidant effects. A Tufts University study found that animals given a flavonoid-enhanced diet had an increase in T-regs and a decrease in Immunoglobulin E (IgE) antibodies—molecules involved in the allergic response.

The flavonoids in tea are particularly helpful. But you'll get healthy amounts from many different plant foods, including onions, blueberries, sweet potatoes, apples and bell peppers.

•**Lots of strawberries.** Strawberries are the richest food source of fisetin, a type of flavonoid that helps preserve T-regs. Fisetin blunts the allergic response and has been shown in laboratory studies to help prevent allergic asthma.

Important: Organic strawberries, fresh or frozen, have more vitamin C and other antioxidants than conventionally grown berries.

•**Put parsley on your plate.** It's more than just a garnish. It's high in apigenin, a flavonoid that decreases the activity of allergy-inducing lymphocytes and reduces levels of IgE. The carotenoids in parsley (it has more than carrots) also are helpful.

•**Eat seafood twice a week (as long as you're not allergic).** A lack of omega-3 fatty acids can cause or aggravate allergy symptoms. People with allergies actually need more of these fats because their cells don't metabolize them efficiently.

•**Broaden your palate.** While tea, parsley and strawberries are among the allergy-fighting stars, all plant foods can help balance the immune system and reduce symptoms. I'm a big fan of legumes (such as black beans, garbanzo beans and lentils), along with carrots, sweet bell peppers, spinach and brussels sprouts. Most of your diet should consist of these and other healthful plant foods.

Hidden Allergy Symptoms

Here are allergy symptoms that aren't typically associated with allergies...
  Anxiety
  Bloating
  Brain fog
  Constipation or Diarrhea
  Depression
  Fatigue
  Headaches
  Insomnia
  Joint pain
  Muscle aches
  Stomachaches
  Weight gain

Foods That Help Stop Seasonal Allergies

Peter J. D'Adamo, ND, director, University of Bridgeport Center of Excellence in Generative Medicine, and distinguished professor of clinical sciences, University of Bridgeport College of Naturopathic Medicine, Bridgeport, Connecticut. He also is the founder of D'Adamo Personalized Nutrition in Wilton, Connecticut, and author of numerous books, including the international best-seller *Eat Right 4 Your Type* and *Allergies: Fight Them with the Blood Type Diet*. DAdamo.com

Seasonal allergies got you sniffling and sneezing? An antihistamine pill would help for a while (though some leave you feeling foggy-brained), but there's an even better solution that doesn't involve taking pills. Instead of heading to your medicine cabinet, head into your kitchen—because certain foods have natural antihistamine effects, a top naturopathic doctor says. Incorporating these foods into your daily diet can help you feel well all through the allergy season, without grogginess or other unwanted side effects.

Why these foods help: When a seasonal allergen enters your body through your eyes, nose or mouth, it upsets the normal routine of cells located in the nasal passages, sinuses, throat and the clear covering of the eyes. In response, those cells release the substance histamine, which triggers the itching, sniffling, sneezing, tearing and other annoying symptoms.

Similar to the way that antihistamine medicines reduce the cells' histamine reaction to allergens, compounds called flavonoids also have antihistamine properties—and you can easily get these flavonoids from your diet.

Allergy-Fighting Flavonoids

Incorporating the following foods into your daily diet can help reduce or eliminate your need for antihistamine medication. For maximum effect, do this year-round, or at least begin two months before your symptoms typically flare up.

Aim for two or more servings per day from each of the following categories. *You're focusing on foods that are rich in...*

•**Anthocyanins.** These flavonoids give dark purple and red foods their characteristic hue. Not only do they act as natural antihistamines, they also have anti-inflammatory properties. This means that anthocyanin-rich foods help reduce swelling in sinuses and nasal passages and relieve the congestion that leads to headaches and trouble sleeping. Good sources include black beans, blackberries, black currants, blood oranges, blueberries, eggplant, elderberries, red cabbage, red leaf lettuce and red onion.

•**Carotenoids.** Among the most widespread groups of naturally occurring pigments, carotenoids are largely responsible for the red, orange and yellow color of various vegetables and fruits, though they also are found in many dark green vegetables and in other foods as well. A study from the Institute of Epidemiology in Germany found that people with high blood levels of carotenoids, reflecting a diet rich in these flavonoids, were at lower risk for allergic rhinitis. To get more carotenoids into your diet, eat apricots, carrots, collard greens, eggs (the yolks contain carotenoids), kale, salmon, spinach, squash, sweet potatoes and tomatoes. Try seasoning foods with cayenne pepper and chili pepper, too, since these spices also provide carotenoids.

•**Quercetin.** A yellowish flavonoid food pigment, quercetin appears to help prevent immune cells from releasing histamine. Good sources include apples, broccoli, capers, citrus fruits, olive oil, onions, parsley, raspberries, red wine and sage.

Also helpful: Green tea. The particular flavonoids in green tea tend to stabilize cells in the body responsible for the release of histamine. In addition, green tea contains theanine, an amino acid that has been shown to block histamine release. Green tea is better at fighting allergies than black or oolong tea because it is less processed and thus retains more of its healthful properties, he added. Drink a cup or more of green tea daily for further relief from aggravating seasonal allergies.

Hidden Food Allergy

Richard Firshein, DO, founder and director of the Firshein Center for Integrative Medicine in New York City. A leading authority in preventive and nutritional medicine that integrates Eastern and Western medical practices, he is the author of *Reversing Asthma* and *The Vitamin Prescription (for life).*

Allergies are a tricky health problem—largely because people tend to self-diagnose based on what they believe to be their allergic trigger. *But that can lead to mix-ups, as allergies, related to those below, go undetected...*

•**Chocolate.** If a piece of chocolate causes symptoms, such as a rash or trouble breathing, the actual culprit may be one of its ingredients, such as soy lecithin, milk or nuts.

What to do: Get checked to see if you're allergic to cocoa, the health-promoting substance in chocolate. If you're not, get further testing to reveal the true source of your allergy, which then can be avoided.

•**Alcohol.** Many people who drink wine, beer and/or hard liquor experience flushed skin, itching, nasal congestion and even an elevated heart rate. For some individuals, protein residues from the alcoholic beverage cause the reaction.

But for many others, the trigger is actually sulfites, chemicals that act as a preservative and prevent the growth of mold or bacteria.

Other examples of foods and drinks that may contain sulfites: Dried fruits...soft drinks...cookies...crackers...noodle or rice mixes...and shellfish.

For a more detailed list, go to: Sulfites.org/sulfite-foods/.

What to do: If testing shows that you are allergic to sulfites, read labels and avoid products that contain this additive. It can also be listed on the label in one of various forms, such as potassium bisulfate...sulfur dioxide...and potassium metabisulfite. Note: Alcoholic beverages also may contain contaminants, such as gluten and yeast, that may require further testing by a doctor.

Best Testing Options

The only way to know for sure that you have an allergy is to undergo allergy testing. If you are truly allergic to something, your immune system mistakes an otherwise harmless substance for an intruder, producing immunoglobulin E (IgE) antibodies. *Two main types of tests identify environmental allergies (such as pollen, dust, mold, etc.) and food allergies (such as peanuts, eggs, soy, milk, etc.)...*

Foods for Better Breathing

A diet high in fiber—especially from fruits and vegetables—can protect against such lung conditions as chronic obstructive pulmonary disease (COPD) and asthma.

New study: Spirometry tests found that among more than 1,900 adults, those who ate the most fiber every day had the best lung function.

Possible reason: Inflammation underlies many lung diseases, and fiber has anti-inflammatory properties. Fiber also changes the composition of the gut microbiome, which may release lung-protective compounds.

Corinne Hanson, PhD, RD, associate professor of medical nutrition, University of Nebraska Medical Center, Omaha.

• **Skin tests.** A suspected allergen is introduced into the body by pricking, scratching or injecting it into the skin—or by applying a skin patch coated with it.

• **Blood tests.** These tests can be used if the doctor is concerned about a dramatic skin reaction that could cause a severe allergic response...or if a person has psoriasis or some other skin condition that could be aggravated by skin testing.

For example, with the radio allergosorbent test (RAST), a sample of your blood is exposed to a suspected allergen.

Note: Sometimes you may not have an actual allergy, but rather a sensitivity that produces allergy-type symptoms when you are exposed to the substance. A separate test is needed to identify an environmental or food sensitivity.

The Right Doctor to See

To get an accurate diagnosis, it's fine to start with a family physician who is well versed in allergies. If you suspect a food allergy, be sure the doctor is experienced in this problem. Other options...

• **Allergists/immunologists may be the best choice for difficult cases.** To find one near you, consult the American Academy of Allergy, Asthma & Immunology, AAAAI.org.

• **Integrative medicine physicians, who identify allergies as an aspect of overall health, are another choice.** To find one near you, check the American Board of Integrative Holistic Medicine website, ABIHM.org, and search "allergy/immunology" in the specialty field.

•**Naturopathic physicians can also be helpful**, especially in offering guidance on diet and the use of supplements (such as butterbur and quercetin). To find a naturopathic physician, consult the American Association of Naturopathic Physicians, Naturopathic.org.

Super Herb Drink for Lung Health

Mike Moreno, MD, physician in charge of primary care and coordinator for new physician education at Kaiser Permanente in San Diego. Dr. Moreno is the author of *The 17 Day Diet*.

When the lungs do not expand and contract normally, or when the tissues are unusually dry, you're more likely to get colds or other infections, including pneumonia. The herb thyme contains thymol, an antioxidant that may help prevent colds, bronchitis and pneumonia and soothe chronic respiratory problems such as asthma, allergies and emphysema.

Simple thing you can do: Add a cup of thyme tea to your daily routine. If you have a chronic or acute respiratory illness, drink two cups of thyme tea daily—one in the morning and one at night.

To make thyme tea: Steep one tablespoon of dried thyme (or two tablespoons of fresh thyme) in two cups of hot water for five minutes, or use thyme tea bags (available at most health-food stores).

If you take a blood thinner: Talk to your doctor before using thyme—it can increase risk for bleeding. Also, if you're allergic to oregano, you're probably allergic to thyme.

Another simple step: Drink at least six to eight eight-ounce glasses of water every day. This helps loosen lung mucus and flushes out irritants, such as bacteria and viruses.

If You Have COPD...Watch What You Eat

Dawn Fielding, RCP, AE-C, a licensed respiratory therapist and certified COPD and Asthma Educator based in West Haven, Utah. She is executive director of the Chronic Lung Alliance, a nonprofit organization involved in education and research related to chronic lung disease. She is also the author of *The COPD Solution*.

Food choices are a surprisingly important factor in controlling COPD symptoms.

Here's why: Breathing is a process that involves the exchange of carbon dioxide (CO_2) and oxygen in the blood.

A person with COPD has a less efficient oxygen-CO_2 exchange process. Anything that increases the amount of CO_2 in blood (whether it's stress or a certain type of food, such as soda or sugary food products) revs up your breathing rate—which worsens COPD.

What to do...

•**Cut back on foods that increase levels of CO_2 in the blood.** The worst offenders are carbonated beverages (even fizzy water)...and anything made with refined sugar or white flour (everything from cakes and cookies to certain breads and pastas).

•**Avoid caffeinated beverages, including coffee, tea and colas.** Caffeine "wakes up" your nervous system, causing your body to work faster, accelerating your breathing rate. Whenever possible, replace soda and other caffeinated beverages with water. Why water? It helps thin mucus secretions and transports nutrients throughout our bodies. For variety, choose flavored waters (such as those infused with lemon or mint).

CHAPTER 5

Superfoods That Help Your Brain

Superfoods for a Super Brain

Mark Hyman, MD, founder of The UltraWellness Center in Lenox, Massachusetts, and author of *The UltraMind Solution.* DrHyman.com

The aging American population is facing a sharp increase in diagnosed cases of dementia. Alzheimer's disease and other forms of dementia affect about 10% of people 65 and older. Among those in their mid-80s and older, up to half have a significant degree of cognitive impairment.

Millions of younger Americans suffer from less obvious mental impairments, including mild memory loss and diminished alertness, as well as brain-related disorders, such as depression and chronic anxiety.

Research clearly shows that some foods can improve mental performance and help prevent long-term damage. *Best choices...*

•**Sardines.** They have two to three times more omega-3 fatty acids than most other fatty fish. Our bodies use omega-3s for the efficient transmission of brain signals. People who don't get enough omega-3s in their diets are more likely to experience learning disabilities, dementia and depression.

Bonus: Omega-3s reduce inflammation and inhibit blood clots, the underlying cause of most strokes.

Fatty fish also are high in choline, a substance used to manufacture one of the main neurotransmitters (acetylcholine) involved in memory.

Recommended: Three cans of sardines a week. Sardines are less likely to accumulate mercury or other toxins than larger fish.

Caution: Many people believe that flaxseed is an adequate substitute for fish. Although it contains alpha-linolenic acid (ALA), a type of omega-3, only about 10% of ALA is converted to docosahexaenoic acid (DHA) or eicosapen-taenoic acid (EPA), the most beneficial forms of omega-3s and the ones that are plentiful in fish oil.

If you don't like sardines, you can take fish oil supplements (1,000 milligrams twice a day).

•**Omega-3 eggs.** They're among the best foods for the brain because they contain folate along with omega-3s and choline. Folate is a B vitamin that's strongly linked to mood and mental performance. A Finnish study of 2,682 men found that those with the lowest dietary intakes of folate were 67% more likely to experience depression than those with adequate amounts.

Recommended: Up to eight eggs a week. Only buy eggs that say "Omega-3" on the label. It means that the chickens were given a fish meal diet. Eggs without this label contain little or no omega-3s.

•**Low-glycemic carbohydrates.** The glycemic index ranks foods according to how quickly they elevate glucose in the blood. Foods with low glycemic ratings include legumes (beans, lentils) and whole-grain breads. They slow the release of sugars into the bloodstream and prevent sharp rises in insulin.

Why it matters: Elevated insulin is associated with dementia. For example, diabetics with elevated insulin in the blood have four times the rate of dementia as people without diabetes. Elevated insulin damages blood vessels as well as neurons. The damage is so pronounced that some researchers call Alzheimer's disease "type 3 diabetes."

Recommended: Always eat natural, minimally processed foods. They're almost always low on the glycemic index. For example, eat apples instead of applesauce...whole-grain bread instead of white bread...or any of the legumes, such as chickpeas, lentils or soybeans.

•**Nuts.** They're among the few plant foods that contain appreciable amounts of omega-3 fatty acids. They also contain antioxidants, which reduce brain and arterial inflammation that can lead to cognitive decline.

Most of the fat in nuts is monounsaturated—it lowers harmful LDL cholesterol without depressing beneficial HDL cholesterol—important for preventing stroke.

Recommended: One to two handfuls daily. Walnuts and macadamia nuts are among the highest in omega-3s, but all nuts are beneficial. Avoid highly salted and roasted nuts (the roasting changes the composition of the oils). Lightly toasted is okay.

•**Cruciferous vegetables, such as broccoli, brussels sprouts, cauliflower and kale.** They contain detoxifying compounds that help the liver eliminate toxins that can damage the hippocampus and other areas of the brain involved in cognition.

Recommended: One cup daily is optimal, but at least four cups a week. Cooked usually is easier to digest than raw.

•**B-12 foods.** Meat, dairy products and seafood are our only source (apart from supplements) of vitamin B-12 in the diet. This nutrient is critical for brain health. A study published in *American Journal of Clinical Nutrition* found that older adults with low levels of vitamin B-12 were more likely to experience rapid cognitive declines. Older adults have the highest risk for B-12 deficiency because the age-related decline in stomach acid impairs its absorption.

Recommended: Two to three daily servings of organic lean meat, low-fat dairy (including yogurt) or seafood.

Also important: I advise everyone to take a multinutrient supplement that includes all of the B vitamins.

•**Green tea.** It's a powerful antioxidant and anti-inflammatory that also stimulates the liver's ability to break down toxins. Research indicates that green tea improves insulin sensitivity—important for preventing diabetes and neuro-damaging increases in insulin.

Recommended: One to two cups daily.

•**Berries, including blueberries, raspberries and strawberries.** The darker the berry, the higher the concentration of antioxidant compounds. In studies at Tufts University, animals fed blueberries showed virtually no oxidative brain damage. They also performed better on cognitive tests than animals given a standard diet.

Recommended: One-half cup daily. Frozen berries contain roughly the same level of protective compounds as fresh berries

Two Tasty Spices for Brain Health

Janet Bond Brill, PhD, RDN, FAND, is a nutrition, health and fitness expert specializing in cardiovascular disease prevention. Dr. Brill is a columnist in *Bottom Line Health* newsletter and is the author of *Blood Pressure DOWN*, *Cholesterol DOWN* and *Prevent a Second Heart Attack*. DrJanet.com

When you think of turmeric and saffron, delicious and flavorful Indian and Spanish dishes probably come to mind. A special perk: These two super spices have been recently proven to have excellent brain health benefits.

Turmeric, the main ingredient in curry powder, has been shown to reduce risk for Alzheimer's disease and brain cancer. And exotic saffron has been shown to have an antidepressant effect and to help fight off brain disease such as Alzheimer's and dementia.

Here's some additional information on these powerful spices—as well as easy and tasty ways to use them in your cooking to boost your brain health...

•**Saffron.** Saffron threads are actually the dried stigmas (the part of the flower that traps pollen) of a particular variety of blue flowering crocus (crocus sativus). Commonly used in the cuisines of India, the Middle East, Spain and Portugal, saffron is the spice that gives dishes from these regions their golden-yellow hue. Also known as "red gold" or the "king of spices," saffron beats out truffles as the most expensive food in the entire world. (Premium saffron sells for approximately $130 per ounce!) Luckily, you need only a few threads of this powerful spice to color and flavor an entire dish. Saffron is available in gourmet food markets and online—1 g costs about $12.

Brain-health benefits: The reddish golden color of saffron indicates that it contains carotenoids—plant pigments such as beta-carotene. These powerful antioxidants help the body fight off brain disease, such as Alzheimer's and dementia, boost immune function and lower inflammation. Other studies suggest that this spice can have an antidepressant effect.

How to use it: Saffron works well in rice dishes...seafood recipes such as paella and bouillabaisse...chicken dishes...and even in some desserts, including cakes and puddings. Remember: The tiniest bit of saffron goes a long way. There's an old saying among chefs that if you can taste the saffron, you've used too much. And just two threads (about 10 mg) have been shown to provide health benefits.

•**Turmeric.** The plant turmeric, or Curcuma longa, is also known as Indian saffron and is a member of the ginger family. Curcumin is the compound in turmeric that's responsible for its health effects and its yellow-orange color.

Turmeric is the primary ingredient of curry powder (other spices in curry powder can include chili powder, coriander, ginger and cumin). Turmeric and curry powder are widely available in grocery stores, but for the greatest brain health benefit, opt for turmeric by itself—a 0.95-ounce bottle of ground turmeric costs about $2.*

*Lead contamination has been found in a few turmeric products. To avoid such possible contaminants, buy spices from large, reputable companies such as McCormick and Spice Islands.

Brain-health benefits: Rich in antioxidants and dietary fiber, turmeric is high in pyridoxine, a B vitamin, as well as potassium and manganese. It has been scientifically shown to disrupt the brain plaques that are the hallmark of Alzheimer's disease and to inhibit the growth of malignant brain tumor cells.

How to use it: Toss a little turmeric into smoothies to add a pop of color and an exotic taste...add a pinch to any soup recipe or roasted vegetables... sprinkle onto scrambled eggs...or add to any rice or chicken dish during cooking. Just a dash is all you need. Researchers have found that consuming curry just a few times monthly is linked to improved cognitive function.

Foods That Fight Memory Loss

Rhoda Au, PhD, associate professor of neurology, Boston University School of Medicine, and director of neuropsychology, Framingham Heart Study.

There's a way to potentially prevent Alzheimer's—a disease that we know frustratingly little about—and it's not some exotic, expensive or potentially dangerous drug. It's actually an affordable, natural component that's found in everyday foods. There's a human study that confirms an association between dietary choline, an amino acid found in eggs and some other foods, and better cognitive performance. The study, from Boston University School of Medicine, appeared in an issue of the *American Journal of Clinical Nutrition*.

Brain Booster

Researchers investigated the dietary habits of 744 women and 647 men ranging from 36 to 83 years of age. None had dementia when the study started. In the early 1990s and then again between 1998 and 2001, participants filled out a questionnaire about their diets—they were asked how often they had eaten particular foods in the past year. After the second questionnaire was given, the researchers performed neuropsychological tests to evaluate the participants' cognitive skills, including verbal memory (remembering a story) and visual memory (remembering images). They also did MRI brain scans to see if there were any tell-tale lesions in the white matter areas called white-matter hyperintensities (WMH). WMH in the brain is considered a marker of vascular disease and is strongly associated with cognitive impairments that precede Alzheimer's disease.

The results: First, this study demonstrated that people who were currently eating the most choline performed better on tests of verbal and visual memory, compared with those who currently had the lowest choline intake. Researchers also found that those who had eaten the highest amounts of choline years earlier (as demonstrated by the first questionnaire) were more likely to have little or no WMH. In other words, eating lots of choline may make your memory sharper, and it also may reduce the risk for damage to the brain and even Alzheimer's disease.

How the Nutrient Protects Your Noggin

According to study coauthor Rhoda Au, PhD, associate professor of neurology at Boston University, this is an observational study, so it doesn't prove cause and effect, but it does show a link between choline and memory. Why? Choline's crucial contribution to cognition, said Dr. Au, may be as a building block for a neurotransmitter called acetylcholine, which is known to help transmit information between neurons faster.

Diet "Dos"

How much choline do you need each day? The recommendation from the Institute of Medicine for men is a daily intake of 550 mg and for women, 425 mg. *The richest food sources are…*

- **3.5 ounces of beef liver**—430 mg

- **One large egg**—126 mg

- **3.5 ounces of salmon**—91 mg

- **3.5 ounces (just under one-half cup) of broccoli, Brussels sprouts, cauliflower or navy beans**—approximately 40 mg.

Other sources of choline include cod, almonds, tofu, milk and peanut butter.

Supplements of choline are available, but high doses (more than 3,500 mg per day for adults over age 18, according to Institute of Medicine) can cause symptoms like vomiting and excessive sweating. So if you want to take a supplement, talk to your doctor first—discuss how much you eat in your diet already so you can figure out whether (and what amount of) a supplement is necessary.

Four Best Brain Foods for Women...
Four Best Brain Foods for Men

Daniel G. Amen, MD, a brain-imaging specialist who is founder, CEO and medical director of Amen Clinics. Based in Newport Beach, California, he is author of more than 30 books, including *Unleash the Power of the Female Brain* and *Change Your Brain, Change Your Life.* AmenClinics.com

Women and men need different foods. *Reason*: They have very different brains.

In a recent study of 46,000 brain scans involving about 26,000 patients, a brain-imaging test called SPECT (single photon emission computed tomography) showed clear differences between male and female brains.

In general: Women's brains are more active than men's brains. Much of this activity is in the region known as the prefrontal cortex, which controls judgment, impulse control and organization. Women also produce less serotonin than men. Serotonin is the neurotransmitter that makes you less worried and more relaxed, so women are more prone to anxiety and depression.

Men, on the other hand, produce less dopamine. Dopamine is involved with focus and impulse control, so men are more likely to be impulsive and have trouble concentrating.

Best Foods for Women

Foods that increase serotonin are critical for women. *When their serotonin levels rise, women naturally experience less anxiety and are less likely to get upset...*

•**Chickpeas.** Also known as garbanzo beans, chickpeas increase the brain's production of serotonin. Other carbohydrates do the same thing, but chickpeas are better because they're high in nutrients and fiber, with about 12 grams of fiber per one-cup serving. Fiber slows the body's absorption of sugars... prevents sharp spikes in insulin...and helps the brain work at optimal levels.

•**Sweet potatoes.** They're my favorite starch because they taste good, are high in vitamin C and fiber and don't raise blood sugar/insulin as quickly as white potatoes. They're a "smart" carbohydrate that causes a gradual increase in serotonin.

•**Blueberries.** They're called "brain berries" for a reason. Blueberries are a concentrated source of flavonoids and other antioxidants that reduce brain inflammation. This is important for good mood and memory. Studies have shown that people who eat blueberries may have less risk for dementia-related cognitive declines.

You will get some of the same benefits with other berries, including strawberries, but blueberries are a better choice for brain function.

●**Dark chocolate.** It is one of the healthiest foods that you can eat. Chocolate increases levels of nitric oxide, a molecule that dilates arteries throughout the body, including those in the brain. One study found that women who ate the most chocolate had greater improvements in verbal fluency and other mental functions than those who ate the least. Chocolate also can improve your mood and energy levels. Because it's high in antioxidants, it reduces the "oxidative stress" that can impair memory and other brain functions.

Best Foods for Men

Men naturally gravitate to high-protein foods. The protein increases dopamine and provides fuel for a man's greater muscle mass. *The trick for men is choosing healthier protein sources…*

●**Salmon.** Between 15% and 20% of the brain's cerebral cortex consists of docosahexaenoic acid (DHA), one of the omega-3 fatty acids found in salmon and other fatty fish such as tuna, trout, sardines, herring and mackerel. Men who don't eat fish are more likely to have brain inflammation that can impair the transmission of nerve signals.

A study published in *Alzheimer's & Dementia: The Journal of the Alzheimer's Association* found that elderly adults who got more DHA had improvements in memory and learning. The study focused on supplements, but you can get plenty of DHA and other omega-3s by eating fatty fish more often.

●**Eggs.** They are not the dietary danger that people once thought. New research has shown that people who eat a few eggs a week—or even as many as one a day—are no more likely to develop heart disease or have a stroke than those who don't eat eggs.

Eggs are an excellent source of protein, inexpensive and easy to prepare. They also are high in vitamin B-12, which can reduce age-related brain shrinkage and improve cognitive function.

●**Sesame seeds and Brazil nuts.** In addition to increasing dopamine, they contain antioxidants that protect brain cells. Like other nuts and seeds, they're high in protein and monounsaturated fats that reduce LDL "bad" cholesterol.

Nuts and seeds are good for the heart as well as the brain. The landmark Adventist Health Study, conducted by researchers at Loma Linda University, found that people who ate nuts five or more times a week were only about half as likely to have a heart attack as those who rarely ate them.

Seven Foods That Make You Smarter

Daniel G. Amen, MD, and Tana Amen, BSN. Dr. Amen ia brain-imaging specialist who is founder, CEO and medical director of Amen Clinics. Based in Newport Beach, California, he is author of more than 30 books, including *Unleash the Power of the Female Brain* and *Change Your Brain, Change Your Life.* His wife, Tana Amen, is a nutritional expert and neurological intensive care nurse. AmenClinics.com

We all know that we need to eat right to keep our minds sharp. But some foods really pack a punch when it comes to memory, learning and other cognitive abilities. *Here, one of America's top brain specialists reveals the seven super brain boosters…*

1. Coconut water. It's high in potassium, a mineral that is critical for brain health. Potassium causes nerve cells to "fire" at the right speed. People who don't get enough potassium tend to have a slower rate of brain activity and may experience confusion and slower reaction times.

Potassium is particularly important if you eat a lot of salt. The body needs to maintain a proper sodium-potassium balance. You should consume roughly twice as much potassium as sodium.

A medium-sized banana has more potassium (about 450 mg) than coconut water (about 250 mg per eight-ounce serving), but bananas also are higher on the glycemic index, a measure of how quickly the food is converted into glucose. The brain works more efficiently when sugars enter the bloodstream gradually rather than "spiking." Coconut water achieves this more readily than bananas.

Recommended: About one cup of coconut water daily. It has a light taste and is low in calories. If you want, you can add it to smoothies or mix it with milk and pour it over breakfast cereals.

2. Blueberries. Sure, blueberries are good for you, but you may not realize just how super rich in inflammation-fighting antioxidants they are. Their oxygen radical absorbance capacity (ORAC, a measure of a food's antioxidant ability) is 2,400, compared with 670 for cherries and 483 for pink grapefruit.

Studies at Tufts University showed that animals that had blueberries added to their diet performed better on cognitive tests than those given a standard diet. They also had increased cell growth in the hippocampus, the part of the brain associated with memory.

Recommended: One-half cup daily. If you don't like blueberries, opt for strawberries or acai berries (a purple, slightly tart berry available in many health-food stores).

Or try Concord grape juice. Researchers from the University of Cincinnati tested Concord grape juice versus a placebo beverage on 21 volunteers, average age 76, suffering from mild cognitive impairment. After 16 weeks, those in the grape-juice group scored better on tests of memory than those drinking the placebo. Also, MRI testing showed greater activation in key parts of the brain, suggesting increased blood flow.

3. Sardines. Salmon often is touted as a healthy fish that is high in omega-3 fatty acids, fats that protect the brain as well as the heart and arteries. Sardines are even better. They also contain generous amounts of omega-3s, but because of their small size, they accumulate lower levels of mercury and other toxins than larger fish.

The membranes that surround brain cells require omega-3s for the efficient transmission of signals. A Danish study that looked at the diets of more than 5,000 adults found that those who ate the most fish were more likely to maintain their memory than those who ate the least. Other research has shown that people who eat fish as little as once a week can lower their risk for dementia.

Recommended: At least two to three servings of fish a week. If you prefer salmon to sardines, be sure to buy wild salmon. It contains more omega-3s than farm-raised fish.

Also helpful: Avocados. They're among the best plant sources of omega-3s.

4. Walnuts. All nuts are good for the brain (as long as they're not roasted in oil and covered with salt). Like fish, nuts are rich in omega-3 fatty acids. They're also loaded with vitamin E, which, in some studies, has been shown to slow the progression of Alzheimer's disease. In addition, nuts reduce LDL "bad" cholesterol (important for preventing stroke). Walnuts are particularly good because they have very high levels of omega-3s. Macadamia nuts are another good choice.

Bonus: The Adventist Health Study, conducted by researchers at Loma Linda University, found that people who ate nuts five or more times a week were about half as likely to have a heart attack as those who rarely ate nuts.

Recommended: About one-quarter cup daily. Nuts are higher in calories than most plant foods, so you don't want to eat too many.

5. Sweet potatoes. They are another low-glycemic food that causes only small fluctuations in blood sugar. This can help you maintain energy and concentration throughout the day. We routinely advise patients to eat sweet potatoes because they satisfy a craving for carbohydrates, and they're also high in beta-carotene and other important antioxidants that keep the brain sharp.

One sweet potato (when you eat the skin) provides more fiber than a bowl of oatmeal. Dietary fiber lowers cholesterol and improves brain circulation.

Recommended: Eat sweet potatoes two to three times a week. If you don't like sweet potatoes, eat yellow squash or spaghetti squash.

6. Green tea. It contains the potent antioxidant epigallocatechin gallate that protects brain cells from free radicals caused by air pollution, toxins, a high-fat diet, etc. Green tea also contains compounds that increase levels of dopamine in the brain. Dopamine is a neurotransmitter that stimulates the brain's reward and pleasure centers and makes you more motivated to make positive lifestyle choices.

Bonus: A double-blind study that looked at patients with mild cognitive impairment found that an amino acid in green tea, L-theanine, improved concentration and energy and reduced anxiety.

Recommended: Two cups daily.

7. Turmeric. The bright yellow color indicates high levels of antioxidants. People who use this spice several times a week have significant reductions in C-reactive protein, a substance that indicates inflammation in the brain and/or other tissues.

A study that looked at more than 1,000 elderly people found that those who ate curry—which includes generous amounts of turmeric—regularly did better on mental-status evaluations than those who rarely or never ate it. All spices with bright, deep colors are high in neuroprotective antioxidants.

Examples: Both ginger and cinnamon appear to have brain-protective properties similar to those of turmeric. And sage improves memory.

Recommended: Add one-quarter teaspoon to one-half teaspoon of any of these spices to your food every day.

Delicious Foods That Prevent Stroke

Roger Bonomo, MD, neurologist in private practice, stroke specialist and former director, Stroke Center, Lenox Hill Hospital, New York City.

According to a recent analysis of seven studies, eating foods that are rich in magnesium may save you from having a stroke. *That includes a list of tasty items that might surprise you...*

A Mighty Mineral

The researchers found seven published studies that analyzed the link between magnesium and stroke risk in a total of 241,000 men and women from the US, Europe and Asia. All studies focused on magnesium intake from food. Researchers determined how many milligrams (mg) of magnesium participants consumed from their self-reports of foods they ate each day.

The results: Magnesium was clearly associated with reduced stroke risk. For every 100 mg of magnesium that study participants consumed each day, their risk for an ischemic (blood clot) stroke went down by about 9%. That's a big drop in risk! And the studies' risk estimates were adjusted for other factors that might affect stroke incidence—including diabetes, body mass index, physical activity levels, high blood pressure, alcohol consumption, age and smoking—so it really does seem to be the magnesium that does the trick.

How might magnesium contribute to such a significant drop in stroke risk? Prior research has indicated that magnesium reduces blood pressure and the risk for diabetes—two prominent risk factors for stroke.

Potassium Lowers Stroke Risk

People who ate at least three pieces of potassium-rich fruit daily had a 21% lower risk for stroke than those who didn't consume that much of the mineral, say researchers from University of Naples Medical School in Italy. When people think of potassium, they usually think of bananas, but prunes and apricots (if dried, look for sulfite-free versions), honeydew melon and cantaloupe also are high in potassium. Eat up!

Mark A. Stengler, NMD, a naturopathic doctor and founder of the Stengler Center for Integrative Medicine in Encinitas, California. He is author or coauthor of numerous books, including *The Natural Physician's Healing Therapies* and *Bottom Line's Prescription for Natural Cures,* and author of the newsletter *Health Revelations.* MarkStengler.com

What's interesting is that among Americans studied, the average daily intake of magnesium from food was only 242 mg—that's less than the 320 mg and 420 mg recommended for women and men, respectively, by the USDA. So even though magnesium appears to be a powerful way to fight off stroke, most Americans aren't getting enough.

You might be wondering if the subjects in these studies were taking multivitamins that may have contained magnesium. Two of the seven studies adjusted for that, while the others didn't. In other words, taking a multivitamin might provide some magnesium, but it might not be enough. Check the bottle to see how much you're getting in your multi...but you'll want to eat magnesium-rich foods as well.

More Magnesium, Please!

Let's recap: Consuming an additional 100 mg of magnesium a day may reduce your risk for stroke by 9%. And magnesium isn't an expensive drug with side effects—it's a natural mineral that's already in many of the foods we eat. So what are you waiting for? Most of us—especially those of us at high risk for stroke, high blood pressure or diabetes—would benefit from eating more magnesium-rich foods, such as...

Pumpkin seeds (191 mg per ¼ cup)

Almonds (160 mg per 2 oz.)

Spinach (156 mg per cup)

Cashews (148 mg per 2 oz.)

White beans (134 mg per cup)

Artichokes (97 mg per one large artichoke)

Brown rice (84 mg per cup)

Shrimp (39 mg per 4 oz.)

You can also supercharge your cooking with magnesium if you use oat bran (221 mg per cup) and buckwheat flour (301 mg per cup).

Should anyone be concerned about overdosing on magnesium? It's hard to eat too much. If we do, our kidneys excrete the extra through urine, so only those with kidney failure need to make sure they don't overdo it with magnesium.

Coffee Protects Against Stroke

Drinking one cup of coffee daily (regular or decaffeinated) reduced risk for stroke by 30%, say researchers from University of Cambridge, England. Consuming more did not yield a greater benefit.

Best: Black coffee because sugar and the fat in milk negate the coffee's anti-inflammatory properties.

Mark A. Stengler, NMD, a naturopathic doctor and founder of the Stengler Center for Integrative Medicine in Encinitas, California. He is author or coauthor of numerous books, including *The Natural Physician's Healing Therapies* and *Bottom Line's Prescription for Natural Cures*, and author of the newsletter *Health Revelations*. MarkStengler.com

Dr. Terry Wahls's Brain-Boosting Diet Helped Her Conquer Multiple Sclerosis— Imagine What It Can Do for You

Terry L. Wahls, MD, internist and clinical professor of medicine at the University of Iowa Carver College of Medicine in Iowa City and president of the Wahls Foundation, which supports research and provides education to the public about managing multiple sclerosis and other chronic diseases. She is the author of *Minding My Mitochondria: How I Overcame Secondary Progressive Multiple Sclerosis and Got Out of My Wheelchair*. TheWahlsFoundation.com

At age 44, I was diagnosed with multiple sclerosis (MS). Three years later, when I became dependent on a wheelchair, my MS was classified as "secondary progressive," meaning that the disease was steadily progressing with no periods of improvement. I kept getting weaker, even though I was receiving widely used treatments for MS including chemotherapy and immune-suppressing medications.

Now: Thanks to the regimen I designed, I haven't needed a wheelchair or even a cane for years. I ride to work on my bicycle, my energy is good and I've stopped taking medication to treat my MS. What happened?

Here's what I credit for my dramatic turnaround—and a description of how it might help you, as well. Because MS is a neurological disease, this program is designed to also help people who are concerned about dementia or Parkinson's disease, have depression or have suffered a traumatic brain injury or stroke.

Finding a Solution

With the help of my medical training, I began poring over the medical literature and designed my own treatment protocol in 2007 based on my theories of what allowed MS to develop and progress.

In people with MS, immune cells damage the myelin sheath, protein and fatty substances that surround nerve cells in the brain and spinal cord. This results in slower nerve signals, which lead to muscle weakness, a lack of balance and muscle coordination, bladder or bowel spasms, blurred vision and other symptoms.

Medications can reduce symptoms, but they don't accelerate nerve signals. As a result, MS patients battle physical and neurological disability—experienced either episodically or in a steady, unrelenting course. The disease often continues to worsen despite therapy. Within 10 years of initial diagnosis, half of MS patients are unable to work because of disabling levels of fatigue, and one-third need a cane, scooter or wheelchair.

After thoroughly reviewing the research, I decided to put myself on a diet that increases the efficiency of mitochondria, units within cells that supply the energy that's needed for nerve activity. Although the effect of diet on MS was unproven, I firmly believed that this was my best hope for fighting MS.

My eating plan was designed to improve the balance of neurotransmitters and supply the mitochondria with the building blocks needed for healthy nerve activity.

My Brain-Health Diet

People who follow this diet typically notice improvements in neurological symptoms within weeks.*

Because natural foods contain a variety of nutrients that can work synergistically, I recommend taking supplements only when you are unable to get the following nutrients in your diet. Be sure to discuss the supplements (and dosages) with your doctor if you take blood-thinning medication—some supplements may have a blood-thinning effect.

In addition to taking such general steps as avoiding sugary and/or processed foods that are low in key nutrients, make sure you get enough...

•**Sulfur vegetables.** Cabbage, kale, collard greens and asparagus are excellent sources of sulfur, which is used by the body to produce gamma-amino-butyric acid (GABA). This "inhibitory" neurotransmitter counteracts the early brain-cell death that can occur if the neurotransmitter glutamate reaches excessive levels.

My advice: Consume three cups of greens each day, including one to three cups of sulfur-rich vegetables daily.

Also: To get other important nutrients, consume one to three cups of brightly colored vegetables or berries each day.

•**Coenzyme Q-10.** Exposure to environmental toxins, such as detergents, pesticide residues and mercury, has been linked to MS and other neurological conditions, such as dementia and Parkinson's disease. Coenzyme Q-10 is

*Consult your doctor before trying the diet and/or supplements described here—especially if you take any medication or have kidney or liver disease.

a fat-soluble compound that helps minimize the effects of these toxins while increasing the amount of energy produced by mitochondria.

Organ meats, such as calf liver and chicken liver, are among the best sources of coenzyme Q-10. I particularly recommend organ meats for older adults because coenzyme Q-10 production declines with age. It's also suppressed by cholesterol-lowering statin drugs.

My advice: Eat organ meats at least once a week. If you don't like organ meats, sardines, herring and rainbow trout are also high in coenzyme Q-10. Coenzyme Q-10 is available in supplement form, too.

•**Omega-3 fatty acids.** The omega-3 fatty acids in cold-water fish, such as salmon and sardines, are used by the body to produce the myelin that insulates brain and spinal cord cells. Myelin is also used to repair damage caused by MS. Omega-3s are concentrated in the brain and are necessary to help prevent depression and cognitive disorders.

My advice: To avoid concern about mercury and other toxins in cold-water fish, such as salmon, get your omega-3s from fish oil supplements that are purified.

Recommended dose: 1 g to 3 g daily.

•**Kelp and algae.** These detoxify the body by binding to heavy metals in the intestine and removing them in the stool.

My advice: Take supplements—one to two 500-mg to 600-mg capsules of kelp and one to four 500-mg capsules of algae daily. Or, as an alternative, add about a tablespoon of powdered algae—different types include Klamath blue green algae, spirulina and chlorella—to morning smoothies.

•**Green tea.** It's high in quercetin, an antioxidant that reduces inflammation. Green tea also changes the molecular structure of fat-soluble toxins and allows them to dissolve in water. This accelerates their excretion from the body.

My advice: Drink several cups of green tea daily.

Best choice: Finely milled Matcha green tea. It has more antioxidants than the typical tea brewed with dried leaves.

Note: Most types of green tea contain caffeine—on average, about 25 mg per cup.

Is This Parkinson's Disease Cure On Your Spice Rack?

Kalipada Pahan, PhD, professor of neurological sciences, Floyd A. Davis Chair of Neurology, Rush University Medical Center, Chicago. His study appeared in the *Journal of Neuroimmune Pharmacology.*

The Bible makes several references to it. The ancient Egyptians used it to preserve their mummies. The ancient Greeks and Romans used it to help them digest their feasts of lamb and wine. We know it's great for diabetes and glycemic control.

And now we find out that this substance fights Parkinson's disease. What is it?

Cinnamon. Besides being a commonly used spice, cinnamon has a long history as a medicine. Medieval physicians used it to treat arthritis, coughing, hoarseness and sore throats. In fact, it was once so valuable, wars were fought over it.

Cinnamon can prevent symptoms of Parkinson's disease that include tremors, slow, jerky movement, stiffness and loss of balance. Or at least cinnamon has this effect in mice acting as experimental models of Parkinson's disease.

Mouse studies often translate to humans when further research is done— so, given how devastating Parkinson's disease can be...and how familiar and safe cinnamon is...these cinnamon studies merit our attention. If these results are repeatable in Parkinson's disease patients, it would represent a remarkable advance in the treatment of this neurodegenerative disease.

The first thing to know is that we are not talking about just any kind of cinnamon, but a specific, authentic kind.

Two types of cinnamon are sold in the United States—Chinese cinnamon (sometimes sold as Saigon cinnamon) and Ceylon cinnamon. Chinese cinnamon, or cassia, is the more common, less expensive type of cinnamon and is what you generally find in supermarkets. You know it—the usual cinnamon powder or that hard, aromatic curl of wood that you plunk into hot apple cider or cocoa. But this is not really "true" cinnamon and does not have its health benefits. Ceylon cinnamon is true cinnamon, and its sticks are softer and flakier than those of Chinese cinnamon. The powder is also lighter and sweeter smelling. There is virtually no way of knowing whether the powdered cinnamon you buy is true cinnamon or cassia or a mix unless it is specifically marked. So even just for general health, keep that in mind the next time you head out to the grocery store to replenish your spice rack—you may need to go to a higher-end market or even order online to get Ceylon cinnamon.

How Does It Work?

Cinnamon is loaded with antioxidants. It may be therapeutic in Parkinson's disease because its antioxidant effects counteract nitric oxide, a free radical that attacks proteins essential to supporting adequate levels of dopamine. Dopamine is the chemical in our brains that not only makes us feel happy and motivated but also controls many of our muscle and limb movements.

It's known that the amount of proteins like DJ-1 and Parkin decrease in the brains of patients with Parkinson's disease. These proteins also decrease in the brains of mice with Parkinson's disease because of nitric oxide production. After the mice ate ground cinnamon, their livers turned the cinnamon into a metabolite called sodium benzoate. Once the sodium benzoate got to the brain, it decreased the production of nitric oxide, which stopped the loss of Parkin and DJ-1, protected brain cells and allowed the mice to move around more normally, with steadier legs and less need for rest and downtime. It's possible that cinnamon could also prevent or lessen the symptoms of other diseases, such as types of palsy and Lewy body dementia, which are also caused by dopamine dysfunction.

How to Use Cinnamon

These findings are potentially great news for people with Parkinson's disease and those who worry that they carry the potential for it in their genes. As it stands, Parkinson's disease patients must rely on drugs, such as levodopa, to replace dopamine, but these drugs neither cure nor change the course of the disease. They only provide temporary relief. Over time, symptoms become increasingly harder to control, and the drugs often have a wide range of serious side effects.

Cinnamon, however, and its metabolite sodium benzoate, could potentially be among the safest approaches to stop the progression of Parkinson's disease once it's diagnosed.

Unless you're allergic to cinnamon, take one teaspoon a day. But don't attempt to just swallow a teaspoon of dry cinnamon powder "straight-up." It will make you gag and could cause you to cough and inhale the powder into your lungs, which is dangerous. Instead, mix cinnamon into food or drink.

You can bet there's much more research coming on cinnamon and Parkinson's—meanwhile, generous helpings of this richly antioxidant spice could be well worth trying.

CHAPTER 6

Superfoods for Your Bones

Dry, Wrinkled Fruit...Strong Bones

Bahram H. Arjmandi, PhD, RD, Margaret A. Sitton Professor and chair, Nutrition, Food, and Exercise Sciences, College of Human Sciences, Florida State University, Tallahassee, Florida.

Prunes...it's not a particularly pleasant word nor a particularly pretty food, but these dark, wrinkly dried fruits are in the process of getting a face-lift. Not only are marketers trying to make prunes more appealing by rebranding them as "dried plums" (which is what they are, of course), but the US Department of Agriculture (USDA) has funded some impressive research that puts muscle behind the makeover, cataloging a long enough list of nutritional benefits that prunes now can be considered a real "superfood." The newest study, from Florida State University, finds that including prunes in your daily diet offers powerful protection against both osteoporosis and bone fracture.

Sweet Protection for Your Bones

Prunes are amazingly good at strengthening bones. Having studied how various fruits, including figs, raisins and strawberries, affect bone health, researchers have found that prunes are uniquely helpful in preventing and/or reversing osteoporosis. That's because they contain compounds that help suppress the natural process of bone breakdown more technically known as resorption—which is a big issue for older people since bone breakdown tends to exceed the rate of new bone growth as people age.

The study spanned one year and involved 236 women who were one to 10 years postmenopausal, either nonsmokers or who smoked 20 cigarettes per day or less, did not have any metabolic diseases and were not taking hormone replacement medication or any other medication that could influence bone health. For the study, half of the women ate 100 grams of prunes (about 10 prunes) each day, while the control group ate 75 grams of dried apple (equal to about two fresh apples, and comparable to the amount of calories, carbohydrates, fat and fiber in 100 grams of prunes). Participants' diets remained the same as normal otherwise. Additionally, everyone in the study took daily doses of calcium (500 milligrams) and vitamin D (400 international units), as do many women.

After a year, a standard bone density X-ray of the ulna (one of two long bones in the forearm) and spine showed that, on average, the women who had been eating the prunes had significantly increased bone mineral density compared with their measured levels before eating prunes. The women who had been eating dried apples, on the other hand, did not lose any bone density during the year of the study, as would have been expected, and their bones showed a slight increase in bone density—indicating that apples are also slightly bone protective, but not to the extent that prunes are. Other bones were measured, but the most dramatic changes were in the ulna and spine—which is gratifying because the ulna and spine are the two major fracture sites linked to osteoporosis.

Learn to Love Prunes

So, what is it about prunes that helps bones? First, they are unusually high in several types of phytonutrients including the antioxidants *neochlorogenic acid* and *chlorogenic acid*, which have been shown to prevent bone loss. Prunes contain larger amounts of boron than most other fruits, and boron helps preserve bone mineral density by modulating bone and calcium metabolism. Prunes also contain iron and potassium, important for blood and heart health.

The women in the study were asked to eat 10 prunes a day, which may be difficult for someone unaccustomed to eating prunes. But eating as few as three prunes a day can have important health benefits. Could all the sugar in prunes cause any problems? The glycemic index of prunes is about 27, among the lowest of all fruits, and none of the women gained any weight during the study (which could be because prunes contain so much fiber). Prunes (unlike other dried fruits) don't contain sulfites—good news for the many folks who are allergic to this common preservative. To prevent mold and yeast spoilage, the preservative potassium sorbate, which is generally regarded as safe and is unlikely to cause allergic reactions, is used. But anyone who wants to avoid it can find prunes that are preservative-free in health-food stores and online.

And what about the laxative effect so often attributed to prunes? They have lots of fiber, including insoluble fiber, which makes them exceptionally good at helping to keep the gastrointestinal (GI) system healthy. Forgetting about the bones for a minute, prunes are really great for digestive health. It's something people may not want to hear about so much, but the truth is, the health of the entire body depends on the health of the GI system. While drinking prune juice certainly can make the bowels move—quickly—eating dried prunes doesn't have the same effect.

Prunes are chewy and sweet but not overwhelmingly sweet like dates, and they have an earthy tartness. Snack on them straight from the box...or chop them up and mix with nuts or add to salads. There are also some really tasty main courses, such as chicken Marbella, that are made with prunes... you can get some unique and delicious recipes by looking online at California Dried Plums Board website, CaliforniaDriedPlums.org

Your Bones Love Carrots and Tomatoes

Katherine L. Tucker, PhD, director, Dietary Assessment and Epidemiology Research Program, Jean Mayer USDA Human Nutrition Research Center on Aging, Tufts University, Boston. Study results were published in the *Journal of Bone and Mineral Research*.

Your list of reasons to eat vegetables may not include bone health—but perhaps it should, now that there's evidence demonstrating that antioxidant pigments in fresh produce protect against bone loss and hip fractures in older people.

Looking at total and individual carotenoid intake over a 17-year period among 370 men and 576 women, average age 75 and all Caucasian, enrolled in the long-term Framingham Osteoporosis Study, investigators found that...

•**People who consumed the most total carotenoids** from foods like tomatoes, carrots, sweet potatoes and cantaloupe experienced a significantly lower risk of hip fractures.

•**Those who consumed the most lycopene**—a carotenoid commonly found in tomatoes and watermelon—likewise had a lower rate of hip fractures and nonvertebral fractures.

•**Beta-carotene**—abundant in carrots, sweet potatoes, mangoes, papayas, etc.—had a small, statistically insignificant protective effect, but only against hip fractures.

Alpha-carotene, beta-cryptoxanthin and lutein plus zeaxanthin did not demonstrate any independent protective effect.

The protective impact of carotenoids is likely derived from their antioxidant activity, as antioxidant pigments block oxidative stress that contributes to bone loss.

Strengthen Bones Naturally Through Diet

The carotenoids most strongly associated with both bone density and reduced fracture risk come from red, orange, yellow and dark green fruits and vegetables. Though some fruits and vegetables are more helpful than others, generally speaking, the more you eat, the better your bones will fare. To strengthen your bones and prevent fractures, eat more than the recommended "Five a Day." Food is preferable over supplements, since it is most likely the synergistic impact of the various polyphenolic compounds and nutrients found in fruits and vegetables that confers the greatest bone protection.

Kale and Osteoporosis

Michael T. Murray, ND, a licensed naturopathic physician based in Paradise Valley, Arizona. Dr. Murray has published more than 30 books, including *Bottom Line's Encyclopedia of Healing Foods,* with coauthor Joseph Pizzorno, ND. DoctorMurray.com

Kale's reputation as the king of veggies is based, in part, on its ability to promote bone health. People often think that milk is a great calcium source, but the absorption of calcium from kale and other leafy greens is actually higher—between 40% to 64%, compared with about 32% from milk.

And that's not all. In addition to being rich in calcium, kale also is an excellent source of vitamin K, a critical nutrient that helps anchor calcium into bone. One cup of raw kale supplies more than 600% of the recommended daily vitamin K intake. If you're concerned about bone health, you should definitely make an effort to eat more kale.

Another benefit: Improved heart health. Kale and other greens, as well as beets and celery, have been found to improve blood pressure and blood flow. While a high intake of fruit and vegetables is associated with healthy blood pressure and reduces risk for heart disease and stroke, kale and cruciferous vegetables are linked to even greater protection.

A good goal: Three to four servings of kale and other greens a week.

Important caveat: In normal amounts, kale is among the healthiest foods you can eat. But some people go overboard. Too much kale, like other cruciferous vegetables, can cause flatulence (gas) for many people. Eating too much raw kale (for example, more than three servings a week) can also interfere with the production of thyroid hormone, leading to the formation of a goiter. And because kale is such a rich source of vitamin K, anyone taking *warfarin* (Coumadin), an important anticlotting drug that interacts with this vitamin, should consult a doctor before eating kale or any leafy greens.

CHAPTER 7

Superfoods That Fight Pain

Ginger, Celery, Oats and Other Foods That Fight Pain

David Grotto, RD, founder and president of Nutrition Housecall, LLC, a consulting firm based in Chicago that provides nutrition communications, lecturing and consulting services as well as personalized, at-home dietary services. He is author of *The Best Things You Can Eat: For Everything from Aches to Zzzz*. DavidGrotto.com

Many of us turn to medications to relieve pain. But research has shown that you can help reduce specific types of pain—and avoid the side effects of drugs—just by choosing the right foods. Here, the common causes of pain and the foods that can help. *Unless otherwise noted, aim to eat the recommended foods daily...*

Osteoarthritis

Osteoarthritis causes pain and inflammation in the joints.

Best foods: Bing cherries, ginger, avocado oil and soybean oil.

A study in *The Journal of Nutrition* found that men and women who supplemented their diets with Bing cherries (about two cups of cherries throughout the day) had an 18% to 25% drop in C-reactive protein, a sign of inflammation. Bing cherries contain flavonoids, plant-based compounds with antioxidant properties that lower inflammation.

Ginger also contains potent anti-inflammatory agents that can reduce joint pain. A double-blind, placebo-controlled study found that 63% of people who consumed ginger daily had less knee pain when walking or standing. I recommend one to two teaspoons of ground fresh ginger every day.

Avocado oil and soybean oil contain avocado soybean unsaponifiables (ASUs), which reduce inflammation and cartilage damage in arthritis patients.

Rheumatoid Arthritis

This autoimmune disease causes systemic inflammation—your joints, your heart and even your lungs may be affected.

Best foods: Fish and vitamin C–rich foods.

The omega-3 fatty acids in fish increase the body's production of inhibitory prostaglandins, substances with anti-inflammatory effects. A recent study found that some patients who consumed fish oil supplements improved so much that they were able to discontinue their use of aspirin, ibuprofen and similar medications.

Ideally, it's best to eat two to three servings of fish a week. Or take a daily fish oil supplement. The usual dose is 1,000 milligrams (mg) to 3,000 mg. Be sure to work with a qualified health professional to determine what supplement regimen is right for you.

Foods rich in vitamin C (citrus fruits, berries, red bell peppers) are effective analgesics because they help decrease joint inflammation. These foods also help protect and repair joint cartilage. A study in *American Journal of Nutrition* found that patients who ate the most vitamin C–rich fruits had 25% lower risk for inflammation.

Gout

Gout is a form of arthritis that causes severe joint pain that can last for days—and that "flares" at unpredictable intervals.

Weight loss—and avoiding refined carbohydrates, such as white bread, commercially prepared baked goods and other processed foods—can help minimize flare-ups. You also should eat foods that reduce uric acid, a metabolic by-product that causes gout.

Best foods: Celery and cherries.

Celery contains the chemical compound 3-n-butylphalide, which reduces the body's production of uric acid. Celery also reduces inflammation.

Both sweet (Bing) and tart (Montmorency) pie cherries contain flavonoids, although the bulk of science supporting the anti-inflammatory and pain-relieving properties of cherries has been done using tart cherries. (An exception is the study that found that Bing cherries relieve osteoarthritis.) It is hard to find fresh tart cherries, so I recommend dried tart cherries or tart cherry juice.

Migraines

These debilitating headaches are believed to be caused by the contraction and dilation of blood vessels in the brain.

Best foods: Oats, coffee and tea.

Oats are high in magnesium, a mineral that helps reduce painful muscle spasms—including those in the muscles that line the arteries. In one study, researchers found that people who took 600 mg of magnesium daily had a 41.6% reduction in the number of migraines over a 12-week period, compared with only a 15.8% reduction in those who took a placebo.

You can get plenty of magnesium by eating high-magnesium foods. A small bowl of cooked oat bran (about one cup), for example, provides more than 20% of the daily value. Other high-magnesium foods include oatmeal, almonds, broccoli and pumpkin seeds.

The caffeine in coffee and tea helps relieve migraine pain. The antioxidants in both beverages also are helpful.

Caution: Consuming too much caffeine—or abruptly giving it up if you are a regular coffee or tea drinker—can increase the frequency and severity of headaches. Limit yourself to a few cups daily.

Muscle Pain

It usually is caused by tension, overuse or an actual injury, such as a strain or sprain. Because tendons and ligaments (the tissues that attach your muscles to your bones) have little circulation, muscle-related pain can be very slow to heal.

Best foods: Tart cherries and rose hip tea.

Eating as few as 20 dried tart cherries can help reduce pain. So can tart cherry juice.

Example: At the Sports and Exercise Science Research Centre at London South Bank University, researchers gave one-ounce servings of tart cherry juice twice daily to athletes who did intense workouts. These athletes regained more of their muscle function more quickly than those who didn't drink the juice. Studies also have shown that the juice can reduce muscle pain after exercise.

Rose hip tea is high in vitamin C, as well as anthocyanins and a substance called galactolipid—all of which have been shown to combat inflammation and may help ease muscle and joint pain. Have several cups daily.

Nerve Pain

Inflammation or injury to a nerve can cause a burning, stabbing pain that is difficult to control with medications. Examples of conditions that cause nerve pain include sciatica (pain along the sciatic nerve from the lower spine down the back of the leg) and neuropathy (nerve damage), a painful complication of diabetes.

Best foods: Turmeric, figs and beans.

Turmeric, a yellow-orange spice that commonly is used in Indian and Asian cooking, is a very effective analgesic. Like ginger, it is an anti-inflammatory that has been shown to reduce pain about as well as ibuprofen—and with none of the side effects.

Both figs and beans—along with whole grains and green leafy vegetables—are rich in B-complex vitamins, which are essential for nerve health. One study, which looked at a form of vitamin B-1, found that patients who took as little as 25 mg four times daily had an improvement in neuropathy. Other B vitamins may have similar effects.

Cherries: The Fruit That Fights Gout

Yuqing Zhang, DSc, professor of medicine and epidemiology at Boston University School of Medicine and lead author of a study on cherry consumption and gout published in *Arthritis & Rheumatism.*

Even if your home-remedy-loving grandma swore that cherries were good for fighting gout, your doctor may have expressed skepticism due to a lack of scientific data. In fact, the FDA issued warning letters to producers of cherry products, cautioning them against making claims of disease-related benefits.

Now, though, there is some evidence lending support to Grannie's stance. But before we talk about the study, let's go over some background.

No-good gout: An excruciating form of arthritis, gout most often affects the joint at the base of the big toe, though it also can affect other parts of the foot or leg. It flares up at unpredictable intervals, causing pain that can linger for days. Men are at higher risk for gout, but women develop this potentially disabling condition, too, especially after menopause.

Gout tends to be a recurrent problem, with attacks occurring when a chemical called uric acid crystallizes within the joint, causing inflammation. Uric acid forms when the body breaks down purines, substances found in some foods and beverages, including dried beans, peas, liver, anchovies and beer.

Since certain foods can trigger flare-ups, researchers set out to determine whether certain other foods could help prevent gout attacks. Among the foods they focused on were cherries, because previous small studies had encouraging results.

Sweet study: Participants included 633 gout sufferers who, for one year, provided information about their flare-ups, diets and other gout risk factors. Then the researchers, noting the dates of each participant's gout attacks, did an analysis of what the person had eaten in the two days prior to the flare-up…and compared that dietary info with various two-day "control periods" that had not preceded a gout attack.

When patients consumed cherries, their risk of suffering a gout attack in the two days that followed was 35% lower than when they did not eat cherries. Generally speaking, the more cherries they ate, the greater the protective effect, with benefits peaking when people ate three servings over a two-day period (one serving equaled 10 to 12 cherries). Consumption of cherry extract produced similar benefits.

Among patients who took the uric acid–lowering medication *allopurinol* (Lopurin, Zyloprim), use of the drug reduced the odds of a gout attack by 53%—but when these patients also consumed cherries, their flare-up risk was reduced by 75%. It is worth noting, however, that the drug can cause stomach upset, diarrhea, painful or bloody urination, eye irritation, vision changes and other potentially serious side effects.

Why cherries work: Cherries are thought to help prevent gout attacks by lowering uric acid levels in the blood and reducing inflammation.

This observational study did not separate out the data on different types of cherries or cherry products—fresh or dried, tart or sweet, juice or extract. So until randomized controlled trials can provide more information, researchers cautioned patients against abandoning their standard gout treatment. In the meantime, though, if you suffer from this toe-torturing ailment, it may be worthwhile to ask your doctor whether cherries should play a part in your gout prevention plan.

The Amazing Pain-Relieving Diet: Ease Your Aches with These Tasty Foods...

Heather Tick, MD, the Gunn-Loke Endowed professor for integrative pain medicine at the University of Washington, Seattle, where she is a clinical associate professor in the department of family medicine and the department of anesthesiology and pain medicine. She is the author of *Holistic Pain Relief: Dr. Tick's Breakthrough Strategies to Manage and Eliminate Pain.*

It's no joke to say that pain really hurts us—because it makes us less productive, less happy and less able to spring back from other conditions. And it leads millions of Americans to a steady intake of dangerous and, in many cases, counterproductive drugs, such as powerful painkillers, antidepressants and narcotics.

Chronic pain (that which lasts for longer than six months) can occur anywhere in the body—in the muscles...joints...head...stomach...bladder...and so on. And though some people find it hard to believe, there are more Americans affected by pain—whether it is from arthritis, headaches, nerve damage or some other condition—than diabetes, heart disease and cancer combined.

What's the answer? Fortunately, there are a variety of highly effective, evidence-based ways to turn your diet into a pain-fighting machine.

Heal Your Digestive Tract

Pain anywhere in the body is almost always accompanied, and made worse, by inflammation. The inflammatory response, which includes the release of pain-causing chemicals, can persist in the body for decades, even when you don't have redness or other visible signs.

Common cause: A damaged mucosa in the innermost lining of the intestines. The damage can be caused by food sensitivities...a poor diet with too much sugar or processed foods...or a bacterial imbalance, among many other factors. A weakened mucosal lining can allow toxic molecules to enter the body, where they then trigger persistent inflammation.

If you suffer from chronic pain—particularly pain that's accompanied by intermittent bouts of constipation and/or diarrhea—your first step should be to heal the damaged intestinal tissue. To do this...

•**Eat a variety of fermented foods.** They are rich in probiotics, which will help the mucosa heal. Most people know that live-culture yogurt is a good source of probiotics...but yogurt alone doesn't supply enough. You can and should get more probiotics by eating one or more daily servings of fermented foods such as sauerkraut or kimchi (Asian pickled cabbage).

Because highly processed fermented foods—such as canned sauerkraut—will not give you the live probiotics you need, select a product that requires refrigeration even in the grocery store. You also can take a probiotic supplement, which is especially important for people who take antibiotics or who don't eat many fermented foods.

•**Cut way back on sugar.** A high- or even moderate-sugar diet, which includes the "simple sugars" in refined carbohydrates such as bread and other baked goods as well as white rice, many breakfast cereals and most juices, increases levels of cytokines, immune cells that cause inflammation.

•**Limit red meat.** Red meat, especially the organic, grass-fed kind, does have valuable nutrients and can be part of a healthy diet. But eaten in excess (more than three ounces daily), red meat increases inflammation. If you eat more than the amount above, cut back. At least half of each meal should be foods grown in the ground—such as vegetables, nuts and seeds. One-quarter should be whole grains, and the rest should be protein, which doesn't always mean animal protein. Other good protein sources include lentils, beans and tempeh.

Eat Other Foods That Turn Off the Fire

Avoiding inflammatory foods is only half the equation—the other half, if you want to reduce pain, is to eat foods that can reduce the inflammation in your body.

If you are expecting an exotic recommendation here, sorry—because what you really need to eat to reduce inflammation in your body is lots and lots of vegetables—raw, steamed, sautéed, baked or roasted. Vegetables contain cellulose, a type of fiber that binds to fats and some inflammatory substances and carries them out of the body in the stools. The antioxidants in vegetables, such as the lycopene in tomatoes and the indole-3-carbinol in crucifers such as broccoli, cabbage and Brussels sprouts, further reduce-inflammation.

This part of your pain-reduction strategy is pretty simple, really: There is not a vegetable on the planet that will worsen your pain…and most of them, if not all, will help reduce your pain. For easy, general dietary guidelines, just follow the well-known, traditional Mediterranean-style diet, which includes lots of vegetables, fish (fish oil is anti-inflammatory), small amounts of red meat and olive oil.

Helpful: It's good to avoid sweets, but make an exception for an ounce or two of dark chocolate daily. Chocolate that contains at least 70% cocoa is very high in antioxidants. It reduces inflammation, improves brain circulation and lowers blood pressure, according to research. And because it's a sweet treat, it will make it easier for you to say "no" to the nasty stuff like cake, cookies and ice cream.

Don't Forget Spices

Turmeric and ginger are great spices for pain relief and can replace salty and sugary flavor enhancers. Ginger tea is a delicious pain fighter. Also, garlic and onions are high in sulphur, which helps in healing.

Coffee: Yes...But

Even though some people can stop a migraine by drinking a cup of coffee when their symptoms first start, too much coffee (the amount varies from person to person) can have a negative effect on other types of pain. It increases the body's output of adrenaline, the stress hormone, as well as inflammation. It also masks fatigue, so you're more likely to push yourself too hard.

Dr. Tick recommends: Do not drink more than one or two cups of coffee daily. I love coffee, but I limit myself to that amount...and I give it up for about a week once every three months. This stops me from getting addicted. Reducing coffee gradually over several days also helps prevent a caffeine-withdrawal headache.

Spices With Surprising Health Benefits

The late **James A. Duke, PhD,** an economic botanist retired from the USDA, where he developed a database on the health benefits of various plants (ARS-grin.gov/duke/). He is the author of numerous books including, most recently, *The Green Pharmacy Guide to Healing Foods: Proven Natural Remedies to Treat and Prevent More Than 80 Common Health Concerns.*

You probably already know that sprinkling cinnamon on your food helps control blood sugar levels and using ginger can ease nausea.

What fewer people realize: There are several lesser-known spices that not only give foods wonderful flavors, but also offer significant health benefits.* In some cases, spices can be just as helpful as medication for people with certain conditions—and safer.

Common medical conditions that you can help prevent—or improve—with the use of spices...

Oregano for Arthritis

Oregano helps alleviate osteoarthritis and other inflammatory conditions, such as rheumatoid arthritis. You might be surprised to learn that this favorite spice of Italian cooking contains natural compounds that have many of the same effects as the powerful anti-inflammatory COX-2 inhibitor drug *celecoxib* (Celebrex).

In addition, oregano contains dozens of other anti-inflammatory compounds that act as muscle relaxants and pain relievers. Unlike celecoxib, which may increase heart attack risk in some people, oregano actually protects the heart by helping to prevent blood clots and irregular heart rhythms.

Best uses: Use oregano liberally on salads or on pizzas. Oregano also can be mixed with peppermint and/or spearmint for a hot or iced mixed-herb tea. If you prefer to take an anti-inflammatory supplement, oregano is one of the half dozen spices in a product called Zyflamend (its ingredients also include rosemary and turmeric). The herbs in Zyflamend act synergistically to provide a more powerful effect than each would when used individually. Zyflamend can be purchased in health-food stores and online. Follow label instructions.

Onion for High Blood Pressure

Onion contains blood-thinning compounds, all of which have a blood pressure–lowering effect. One of the most potent of these compounds is the flavonoid quercetin. Onion also acts as a natural diuretic, which lowers blood pressure by helping the body excrete excess fluids and salt.

Fish Eases Arthritis

Eating fish has many health benefits, including reducing inflammation.

New finding: In a study of the diets of 176 patients with rheumatoid arthritis, those who ate non–fried fish two or more times a week had less rheumatoid arthritis activity—as measured by a combination of swollen and tender joints and a blood marker for inflammation—than those who ate fish once a month or never.

Sara K. Tedeschi, MD, MPH, rheumatologist, Brigham and Women's Hospital, Boston.

---

*Check with your doctor before using any of the spices mentioned in this article for medicinal purposes. The natural compounds found in spices may interact with some prescription drugs. Pregnant and nursing women should avoid using spices medicinally.

Best uses: If possible, use a full onion (all types contain some blood pressure–lowering compounds) in onion soup, for example.

Reason: The onion's thin outer skin is the plant's best source of quercetin. Onion powder and cooked onions are not as effective as fresh onion.

Research shows that people who take quercetin as a supplement can lower their blood pressure in less than a month. In a 2007 double-blind study, people with hypertension who took 730 mg of quercetin daily for 28 days lowered their systolic (top number) blood pressure by an average of 7 mm HG and diastolic (bottom number) by 5 mm HG.

Fennel Seed for Indigestion

Fennel seed is surprisingly effective at relieving indigestion. If I get indigestion, I pick some fennel seeds from the fennel plant in my garden. Fennel is easy to grow, and it keeps coming back year after year. In my experience, it can settle the stomach as well as many over-the-counter products.

Fennel seed relaxes the smooth muscles that line the digestive tract, relieving flatulence, bloating and gas, as well as nausea and vomiting, motion sickness and abdominal pain. If you don't want to grow your own, store-bought fennel seed also works well.

Best uses: Fennel seed can be eaten whole (it tastes and smells similar to anise) or made into a tea by pouring boiling water over it (use one gram to three grams of fennel seed—about one-half to one and one-half teaspoons— per cup). To sweeten the tea, molasses or honey is the best choice.

Caution: Because fennel seed can increase estrogen levels, it should be avoided by women who are pregnant or breast-feeding or who have an estrogen-sensitive medical condition, such as estrogen-responsive breast cancer.

The Fruit That Gives Muscle Pain the Boot

Muscle soreness is the big downside of working out.

Good news: When athletes drank 16 ounces of watermelon juice an hour before exercise, they had less muscle soreness than when they did not drink it.

Theory: Watermelon contains L-citrulline, an amino acid that boosts blood flow and oxygen in muscles, reducing pain.

To ease sore muscles: Try eating some watermelon (or drinking the juice if you have a juicer).

Encarna Aguayo, PhD, associate professor of food technology, Technical University of Cartagena, Spain.

Garlic for the Common Cold

While the research on garlic's positive effect on cardiovascular health is perhaps most widely known, this popular allium also boosts immunity, helping to prevent and treat the common cold.

In one study of nearly 150 people who took a garlic supplement or placebo for 12 weeks during cold season, those taking the garlic had significantly fewer colds (or symptoms that eased more quickly in cold sufferers) than those taking a placebo.

Best uses: To help cure or prevent a cold, add a clove or two of garlic to all soups…sprinkle garlic powder on toast…and/or mix diced raw garlic with olive oil and vinegar.

Saffron for Depression

Saffron, a spice derived from a small, blue crocus, acts as a potent antidepressant and has been used for centuries in traditional medicine for this purpose. No one is sure how it works, but its active ingredient, crocetin, appears to enhance blood flow to the brain.

Research conducted in Iran has shown that 30 mg per day of saffron powder (about one-tenth of a teaspoon) relieved mild-to-moderate depression as effectively as standard doses of the antidepressant medications *fluoxetine* (Prozac) and *imipramine* (Tofranil).

Best uses: One of the world's most expensive spices, saffron can be used in herbal tea or chicken paella. A five-gram bottle of Exir Pure Saffron Powder is $32 at Amazon.com.

Golden Milk for Pain Relief

Heather Tick, MD, who holds the Gunn-Loke Endowed Professorship for Integrative Pain Medicine at the University of Washington in Seattle and is a clinical associate professor in both the departments of family medicine, and anesthesiology and pain medicine. She is the author of *Holistic Pain Relief*.

Turmeric, a mildly bitter spice, is a powerful analgesic with impressive anti-inflammatory powers. A 2014 study suggested it may be as effective as ibuprofen in reducing the pain of knee osteoarthritis.

Capsules are one option to try. But if you like the taste, try making "Golden Milk."

What to do: Combine one-quarter cup of turmeric with one-half cup of water in a pot, and blend to create a thick paste. Heat gently, adding a pinch of ground black pepper and drizzling in water as needed to maintain a thick but stirrable consistency.

Refrigerate the mixture in a glass container, and add one heaping teaspoon to an eight-ounce glass of warm water mixed with a little almond milk every day. You can add some honey to cut the bitterness. Or use warm broth instead of water and a dash of ginger and/or garlic for a tasty soup.

*Consult your doctor before trying the home remedy described here—especially if you take blood thinners or have a chronic medical condition such as hypertension.

Cherry Juice for Sore Muscles

Mark A. Stengler, NMD, a naturopathic doctor and founder of the Stengler Center for Integrative Medicine in Encinitas, California. He is author or coauthor of numerous books, including *The Natural Physician's Healing Therapies* and *Bottom Line's Prescription for Natural Cures,* and author of the newsletter *Health Revelations.* MarkStengler.com

When you exercise, particularly after taking time off, your muscles complain—they feel tight, they ache, they make it hard for you to move. As long as there is no actual pain, these are simply signs that your muscles are working...helping you to get fit and burning fat and calories.

You can take a warm bath or, better still, have a massage. And there's something else you can do—drink cherry juice. It has been used for centuries to relieve pain from gout and arthritis, and today some athletes have begun to drink it after working out.

One small study reinforces the effectiveness of this simple treatment. Researchers from the University of Vermont and New York City's Nicholas Institute of Sports Medicine and Athletic Trauma asked 14 male college students to drink 12 ounces of cherry juice or a cherry-flavored placebo drink twice daily for eight days. On the fourth day, participants performed arm-curl exercises. Those who drank cherry juice experienced significantly less pain, soreness and loss of muscle strength.

Cherries are a rich source of anthocyanins—pigments that give cherries their rich color and have potent antioxidant and anti-inflammatory properties. They block enzymes known as COX-1 and COX-2, which are involved in pain and inflammation pathways.

Best choice: Tart cherries, which contain more anthocyanins than sweet cherries. You can buy tart cherry juice in natural-food stores.

Good brands: FruitFast ($24.95 for concentrate to make two gallons of juice) and Cheribundi ($27 for 12 eight-ounce bottles). I recommend drinking up to 24 ounces daily, especially when exercising heavily.

Note: Diabetics should watch sugar content because cherry juice is high in natural sugar.

Super-Broth for Super-Health and Pain Relief

Sally Fallon Morell, founding president of The Weston A. Price Foundation, which champions nourishing, traditional foods such as bone broths, sourdough breads and soaked grains and meat, organ meats and butter and dairy products from grass-fed animals. Based in Brandywine, Maryland, she is author of the best-selling *Nourishing Traditions* and coauthor of *Eat Fat Lose Fat, The Nourishing Traditions Book of Baby & Child Care* and, most recently, *Nourishing Broth: An Old-Fashioned Remedy for the Modern World.* NourishingTraditions.com

Before the 20th century, almost all soups and stews were made with a stock of bone broth—bones and other animal parts slowly simmered in a cauldron or stockpot, producing a nutrient-rich concoction.

Fast-forward to the 21st century, when food processing has largely replaced home cooking. Today's processed "broth" often is nothing more than a powder or cube dissolved in water and spiked with additives such as MSG that mimic the taste of broth.

The loss of bone broth is a big loss.

What most people don't realize: Traditional bone broth delivers unique, health-giving components that can be hard to find anywhere else in the diet. And a brothless diet may be hurting your health—contributing to arthritis, nagging injuries, indigestion and premature aging.

Good news: Bone broth is simple to make or buy. The optimal "dose" is one cup daily. If you are trying to heal, increase this to two cups.

Super-Healthy Ingredients

Bone broth, whether it's made from the bones of a chicken, cow, lamb, pig or the like, is extraordinarily rich in the following...

•**Collagen.** The number-one health-giving component of bone broth is melted collagen, or gelatin. Collagen is the most abundant protein in the body, providing strength and structure to tissue. In fact, microscopic cables of collagen literally hold your body together—in joints, tendons, ligaments, muscles, skin and membranes around internal organs.

Your body makes its own collagen, of course. But it becomes harder for your body to make it as you age, leading to arthritis, wrinkled skin and other degenerative conditions.

•**Glucosamine and chondroitin sulfate.** These two nutrients are well-known for helping to ease arthritis pain—and bone broth supplies ample amounts of both.

Glucosamine is created from glucose (sugar) and glutamine (an amino acid, a building block of protein). It's found in cartilage, the part of the joint that provides cushioning and lubrication between bones.

Chondroitin sulfate is a proteoglycan, a type of molecule that helps hydrate cells. It also supplies sulfur, a mineral that nourishes cartilage and balances blood sugar.

•**Glycine.** This amino acid supports the health of blood cells, generates cellular energy, aids in the digestion of fats, speeds wound healing and helps the body rid itself of toxins, such as mercury, lead, cadmium and pesticides. Glycine also regulates dopamine levels, thereby easing anxiety, depression and irritability and improving sleep and memory.

•**Glutamine.** This amino acid nourishes the lining of the gut, aiding the absorption of nutrients. It boosts the strength of the immune system. It helps the body recover from injuries such as burns, wounds and surgery. It also strengthens the liver, helping the body process and expel toxins. And glutamine boosts metabolism and cuts cravings for sugar and carbohydrates, aiding weight loss.

Feel-Better Broth

Bone broth delivers extra-high levels of all those health-giving compounds, so it's not surprising that it can help prevent and heal many health problems, including...

•**Arthritis and joint pain.** By supplying collagen, glucosamine, chondroitin and other cartilage-nourishing factors, bone broth can repair and rebuild cartilage, preventing osteoarthritis or easing arthritis pain. In fact, bone broth might be the best food for osteoarthritis, which affects more than 30 million Americans.

Compelling research: In a review of seven studies on osteoarthritis and melted collagen (collagen hydrolysate), researchers at University of Illinois College of Medicine in Chicago found that ingesting the compound helped create new cartilage, thus lessening pain and improving everyday functioning.

•**Digestive problems.** In the 19th century, broth and gelatin were widely prescribed—by Florence Nightingale and many others—for convalescents who lacked the strength to digest and assimilate food properly.

Sadly, nutritional therapy for digestive problems went out of fashion after World War II, replaced by pharmaceuticals.

Example: A form of gelatin (gelatin tannate, or Tasectan) is being used as a digestive drug, with studies showing that it can help heal gastroenteritis (stomach and intestinal irritation). The new drug is being hailed as a "gut barrier protector"—but wouldn't it be better to prevent digestive diseases by strengthening your gut with bone broth?

•**Injuries and wounds.** The components in bone broth are crucial for healing broken bones, muscle injuries, burns and wounds—a key benefit for seniors, whose injuries can take longer to heal.

The use of cartilage (a main component of bone broth) for wound healing was championed by John F. Prudden, MD, whose published papers include "The Clinical Acceleration of Healing with a Cartilage Preparation," in the May 3, 1965 issue of *JAMA*. In his research, Dr. Prudden showed that cow cartilage could speed wound healing, produce stronger healing that was less likely to be reinjured and produce smoother, flatter and more natural-looking scars.

More recently, studies have shown that bone broth ingredients—particularly glycine and other amino acids—are uniquely effective at healing wounds, including hard-to-heal diabetic foot ulcers.

•**Infections.** Chicken soup—"Jewish penicillin"—is a classic home remedy for a cold, flu, pneumonia and other infectious diseases. Over the years, researchers studying broth and its components have noted their ability to strengthen immune cells, fight off viruses and calm down the overactive immune system caused by autoimmune diseases such as rheumatoid arthritis, Crohn's disease and psoriasis.

How to Make Bone Broth (or Buy It)

Making a very healthful and delicious bone broth may seem daunting—but it's not. Here's a simple way to make a chicken bone broth. You can use the same method for any kind of animal bones. Beef bones (such as rib bones, short ribs and beef shanks) should be browned first in the oven for the best flavor.

How to prepare bone broth: Whenever you eat chicken, save the bones. You can save skin and meat, too—the skin is rich in collagen, and there is some collagen in the meat. Just put all these leftovers in a zipper freezer bag, and store in the freezer until you have enough to fill a standard six-to-seven-quart slow cooker, about six to eight cups. Add a splash of vinegar and one sliced onion. Fill up the slow cooker with filtered water.

Slow-cook on low overnight. (If you don't have a slow cooker, you can make the broth by simmering it all day in a stock pot.)

In the morning, ladle the broth through a strainer and put the broth in the refrigerator. Fill up the slow cooker with water, and cook the bones again overnight, producing a second batch. As with the first batch, ladle the broth through a strainer. You now have about one gallon of chicken broth, which you can refrigerate or freeze.

What to look for: A sign that your broth is rich in collagen is that it gels when chilled. To get a good gel, it is helpful to add chicken feet or a pig's foot to the bone mix.

You can use your broth as a basic ingredient in soups, stews, sauces and gravies. Or just add a little salt, heat it and drink it in a mug. Try this simple Thai soup: Two cups of chicken broth with one can of coconut milk, the juice of one lime and a pinch of red pepper flakes.

If you want to purchase healthful bone broth, good sources include Bare Bones Broth Company (BareBonesBroth.com), OssoGood (OssoGoodBones. com), Stock Options (StockOptionsOnline.com) and the Brothery (BoneBroth. com). These broths are available by mail order, but you may be able to find them in some gourmet and specialty shops.

Yummy Healing Soups

Sharon Palmer, RDN, registered dietitian and author of *Plant-Powered for Life* and *The Plant-Powered Diet*. She is the editor of the *Environmental Nutrition* newsletter and nutrition editor for *Today's Dietitian*. Her recipes, including those in this article, appear on her website, SharonPalmer.com.

Few foods are more comforting than a piping hot bowl of delicious soup.

What you may not realize: Certain homemade soups are packed with healing nutrients that help fight chronic health problems, including diabetes, arthritis and stomach troubles.

What's so special about soup? With most cooking methods, such as steaming or boiling, the liquid is discarded—along with vitamins and minerals that may have leached out of the food. Not so with soup, which uses all the liquid so that most of the nutrients are preserved, even when heated.

Bonus: Because soups are so filling and satisfying, they have also been shown to help reduce one's overall calorie intake when added to a meal!

My three favorite healing soups —and their "souper" star nutrients (each recipe below makes about four servings)...

For Diabetes Prevention

CURRIED LENTIL QUINOA SOUP

Souper star nutrient: **Fiber.** Diets rich in whole grains, pulses (which include beans, lentils, peas) and vegetables help protect against diabetes. The all-important common denominator in these foods is fiber, which takes longer to metabolize than processed carbs. For this reason, fiber is linked to improved blood sugar control—in people with diabetes and those without the disease.

There's also good news from a 2016 study that found a link between regular consumption of pulses and a healthy body weight—a crucial factor in controlling diabetes.

To get an adequate amount of fiber, the American Diabetes Association recommends that women consume at least 25 g daily...men need a minimum of 38 g. (These amounts are based on average daily calories consumed by women and men.) One serving of this soup provides 20 g of fiber. *Makes about four servings.*

8 cups of water
1½ cups of green lentils (rinse first)
1 cup of rainbow quinoa (rinse first)
1 onion, diced
1 sweet potato, peeled and diced
1 cup of frozen peas
2 medium carrots, sliced
1 cube of vegetable bouillon base
1 cup of tomato sauce
1 tablespoon of tikka masala spice blend*
3 garlic cloves, minced

Instructions: Place the ingredients in a large pot, stir well and cover.

Bring to a boil, then reduce to a simmer, stirring occasionally, for 40 minutes.

*I buy tikka masala spice blend at Seattle's World Spice Merchants...or you can find garam masala (a good substitute for tikka masala spice blend) at most supermarkets.

For Arthritis Prevention

CARNIVAL SQUASH SOUP

Souper star nutrient: **Turmeric.** Traditionally used in Chinese and Indian Ayurvedic medicine to treat arthritis, turmeric contains a powerful chemical called curcumin, which is known to block inflammatory enzymes and proteins.

Instructions: Halve one carnival squash (a somewhat sweeter squash than butternut and available at most supermarkets), scoop out the seeds and slice into quarters, leaving the peel on. Place in a medium pot, add water to cover and cook 20 minutes, until the flesh is tender.

While the squash cooks, sauté three celery stalks, diced…one shallot, diced…and one chopped garlic clove in one teaspoon of olive oil in a skillet. Peel a three-inch segment of turmeric root and slice three-quarters of it into thin slices, reserving the rest for garnish. (Or use three teaspoons of turmeric powder.) Add to the skillet and sauté with vegetables until soft, about 10 minutes.

When the squash is tender, drain the water from the pot and let it cool slightly. Scoop out the flesh and add to a blender with the cooked celery mixture plus one cup each of vegetable broth and plain, unsweetened coconut, soy or almond milk. Blend until smooth, then return to the pot and reheat just until bubbly and heated through. (For easier cleanup, you can blend in the pot with an immersion blender.)

Ladle into bowls, garnishing with grated (or powdered) turmeric and sliced celery leaves.

For Digestive Health

MISO KABOCHA SOUP

Souper star nutrient: **Probiotics.** Trillions of microorganisms reside in your bowels—and that's a good thing! These healthy bacteria, called probiotics, aid digestion and nutrient absorption…govern the immune system…and work to keep harmful pathogens in check.

Emerging research has linked the consumption of probiotics and probiotic-rich foods, such as miso (a traditional Japanese fermented soybean paste), sauerkraut, kimchi, yogurt and kefir, with potential health benefits, including improved immune and digestive function.

Miso is intensely flavorful and provides a note of umami—that is, a meaty, savory taste. This recipe also contains ginger, which helps fight inflammation and nausea.

Instructions: Slice a small, unpeeled kabocha squash (a round green Japanese vegetable available at farmers' markets and an increasing number of supermarkets) into large pieces. Scoop out the seeds, place in a baking dish with a small amount of water and bake at 350°F for 35 minutes (or you can microwave it with a little water for 10 minutes).

Once slightly cooled, scoop out the flesh and place it in a blender with one cup of vegetable broth...one cup of plain, unsweetened coconut, soy or almond milk...one-and-one-half tablespoons of white miso...and one teaspoon of grated fresh ginger. Process until smooth (use an immersion blender in a pot if you prefer). Heat the mixture in a medium pot until bubbly. Stir in one 14-ounce package of tofu (diced in small cubes) and one-half cup of green onions, diced. Delicious!

Healing Herbs and Food for Psoriasis

Jamison Starbuck, ND, is a naturopathic physician in family practice and writer and producer of Dr. Starbuck's Health Tips for Kids, a weekly program on Montana Public Radio, MTPR.org, both in Missoula. She is a past president of the American Association of Naturopathic Physicians and a contributing editor to *The Alternative Advisor: The Complete Guide to Natural Therapies and Alternative Treatments.* DrJamisonStarbuck.com

Psoriasis is difficult to treat. Affecting about 2% of the population, the condition is an overproduction of new skin cells. It shows up on people as thick, red patches covered with silvery, scaly skin. The affected skin tends to flake off, leaving little pieces of skin on the sufferer's clothing and bedding. Psoriasis is uncomfortable because the skin itches and feels tight. Even though the condition is not contagious, it is unsightly and often makes those who have it embarrassed by their skin. Few people realize that psoriasis is in part a genetic condition. However, it may never show up...or a variety of factors—such as hormone changes, poor diet, a hectic lifestyle or medications, including some antibiotics—can stress the body and trigger its onset.

Conventional medicine relies on steroids and immune-suppressive medications to treat psoriasis. These drugs don't cure psoriasis and can have a variety of side effects, including high blood pressure, elevated cholesterol and a weakened immune system. While these drugs are sometimes necessary, nondrug approaches can be used by themselves or in conjunction with pharmaceutical treatment. *What I recommend…**

●**Watch your diet.** Since inflammation fuels psoriasis, people with the condition should eat an anti-inflammatory diet. This means avoiding any food to which you are allergic, which triggers inflammation, as well as sugar, alcohol, processed foods, fast foods and fried foods. Eat a diet rich in vegetables, whole grains, fruits and legumes. Eat no more than six ounces of meat each day, and drink lots of water so waste can be eliminated via the kidneys and stool instead of the skin. When waste is eliminated via the skin, it worsens psoriasis. To boost immune health, consume at least 2,000 mg of flax oil daily—use it in food or take in capsule form. Flax is very high in omega-3 fatty acids, the best type of fatty acid for reducing inflammation. If flax bothers your stomach, try fish oil.

Important: Never cook with flax oil, and do not use it to bake—when heated, flax oil releases harmful free radicals.

●**Try herbs.** Certain herbs have anti-inflammatory properties and promote skin health—both important for psoriasis treatment. I recommend a combination of burdock, cleavers, sarsaparilla and yellow dock. If possible, purchase tinctures of each one of these herbs. Combine equal parts of each in one bottle and take one-quarter teaspoon of the combination, in two ounces of water, twice daily at least 15 minutes before meals.

●**Don't forget topical therapies.** Herbal medicines used topically won't cure psoriasis, but they can ease symptoms. I recommend salves made from calendula, which promotes new skin growth, and comfrey to moisten flaky skin. Look for a product in a base of olive oil and beeswax. Some of these salves, such as All Purpose Salve available from Wise Woman Herbals, also contain vitamin E oil, which has its own healing properties for the skin. Apply several times a day as needed.

My natural medicine protocol can take a couple months to work well. But it's definitely worth trying before resorting to risky drug therapy.

*If you use any prescription medication, have a chronic medical condition or are pregnant or nursing, consult your doctor before using flax oil and/or any herbs. Avoid yellow dock and sarsaparilla if you take *digoxin* (Lanoxin) or diuretics. Calendula and comfrey ointments should not be used on open wounds.

Best Food for Stomach Pain

David Grotto, RD, LDN, a registered dietitian and founder and president of Nutrition Housecall, LLC, a Chicago-based nutrition consulting firm. He is author of *The Best Things You Can Eat.* DavidGrotto.com

Maybe you ate too much…or life's stresses affect your stomach first. You could take an antacid, but it doesn't always help and often causes side effects, including constipation or diarrhea.

Best food: Hot peppers. You wouldn't think that tongue-torching hot peppers would be good for your insides, but they are. They contain capsaicin, a proven pain reliever that works on the inside as well as externally.

One study, which looked at 30 patients with dyspepsia (stomach upset), found that those who consumed about one-half teaspoon of dried red pepper daily for five weeks had a 60% reduction in symptoms. Hot peppers also seemed to help with heartburn.

What to do: To help prevent stomach trouble, eat meals daily that contain "heat"—from chili powder, hot peppers, hot curry and the like. Or add a small amount of cayenne pepper to hot water for a spicy tea.

CHAPTER 8

Superfoods for Better Blood Sugar

Foods That Fight Diabetes and Prediabetes

Bill Gottlieb, CHC, is a certified health coach and health journalist. He is the author or coauthor of numerous books, including *Bottom Line's Speed Healing*. BillGottlieb Health.com

Scientific research and the experience of doctors and other health professionals show superfoods can be even more effective than drugs when it comes to preventing and treating diabetes. I reviewed thousands of scientific studies and talked to more than 60 health professionals about these glucose-controlling natural remedies.

Here are two standout natural remedies...

Caution: If you are taking insulin or other medications to control diabetes, talk to your doctor before changing your diet.

Apple Cider Vinegar

Numerous studies have proved that apple cider vinegar works to control type 2 diabetes. Several of the studies were conducted by Carol Johnston, PhD, RD, a professor of nutrition at Arizona State University.

Standout scientific research: Dr. Johnston's studies showed that an intake of apple cider vinegar with a meal lowered insulin resistance (the inability of cells to use insulin) by an average of 64% in people with prediabetes and type 2 diabetes...improved insulin sensitivity (the ability of cells to use insulin) by up to 34%...and lowered postmeal spikes in blood sugar by an average of 20%. Research conducted in Greece, Sweden, Japan and the Middle East has confirmed many of Dr. Johnston's findings.

How it works: The acetic acid in vinegar—the compound that gives vinegar its tart flavor and pungent odor—blunts the activity of disaccharidase enzymes that help break down the type of carbohydrates found in starchy foods such as potatoes, rice, bread and pasta. As a result, those foods are digested and absorbed more slowly, lowering blood glucose and insulin levels.

Suggested daily intake: Two tablespoons right before or early in the meal. (More is not more effective.)

If you're using vinegar in a salad dressing, the ideal ratio for blood sugar control is two tablespoons of vinegar to one tablespoon of oil. Eat the salad early in the meal so that it disrupts the carb-digesting enzymes before they get a chance to work. Or dip premeal whole-grain bread in a vinaigrette dressing.

Soy Foods

A 10-year study published in *Journal of the American Society of Nephrology* found that the mortality rate for people with diabetes and kidney disease was more than 31%. Statistically, that makes kidney disease the number-one risk factor for death in people with diabetes.

Fortunately, researchers have found that there is a simple way to counter kidney disease in diabetes—eat more soy foods.

Standout scientific research: Dozens of scientific studies show that soy is a nutritional ally for diabetes patients with kidney disease. But the best and most recent of these studies, published in *Diabetes Care*, shows that eating lots of soy can help reverse signs of kidney disease, reduce risk factors for heart disease—and reduce blood sugar, too.

The study involved 41 diabetes patients with kidney disease, divided into two groups. One group ate a diet with protein from 70% animal and 30% vegetable sources. The other group ate a diet with protein from 35% animal sources, 35% textured soy protein and 30% vegetable proteins. After four years, those eating the soy-rich diet had lower levels of several biomarkers for kidney disease. (In another, smaller experiment, the same researchers found that soy improved biomarkers for kidney disease in just seven weeks.) In fact, the health of the participants' kidneys actually improved, a finding that surprised the researchers, since diabetic nephropathy (diabetes-caused kidney disease) is considered to be a progressive, irreversible disease.

Those eating soy also had lower fasting blood sugar, lower LDL cholesterol, lower total cholesterol, lower triglycerides and lower C-reactive protein, a bio-marker for chronic inflammation.

How it works: Substituting soy for animal protein may ease stress on the delicate filters of the kidneys. Soy itself also stops the overproduction of cells in the kidney that clog the filters...boosts the production of nitric oxide, which improves blood flow in the kidneys...and normalizes the movement of minerals within the kidneys, thus improving filtration.

Suggested daily intake: The diabetes patients in the study ate 16 grams of soy protein daily.

Examples: Four ounces of tofu provide 13 grams of soy protein...one soy burger, 13 grams...one-quarter cup of soy nuts, 11 grams...one-half cup of shelled edamame (edible soybeans in the pod), 11 grams...one cup of soy milk, 6 grams.

What's Wrong with Diabetes Drugs?

Doctors typically try to control high blood sugar with a glucose-lowering medication such as *metformin* (Glucophage), a drug most experts consider safe. But other diabetes drugs may not be safe.

Example #1: Recent studies show that *sitagliptin* (Januvia) and *exenatide* (Byetta) double the risk for hospitalization for pancreatitis (inflamed pancreas) and triple the risk for pancreatic cancer.

Example #2: *Pioglitazone* (Actos) can triple the risk for eye problems and vision loss, double the risk for bone fractures in women and double the risk for bladder cancer.

Best Food for Hypoglycemia

David Grotto, RD, LDN, a registered dietitian and founder and president of Nutrition Housecall, LLC, a Chicago-based nutrition consulting firm. He is author of *The Best Things You Can Eat*. DavidGrotto.com

This is a dangerous condition commonly associated with diabetes in which blood sugar levels fall below 70 mg/dL. It can happen periodically to some people with diabetes when the drugs used to treat the condition, such as insulin, work too well and cause an excessive drop in blood sugar.

Best food: Apricots. Seven to eight dried apricot halves provide 15 grams of a fast-acting carbohydrate when you have a crash in blood sugar. Fresh apricots also will help, but the carbohydrates (sugars) aren't as concentrated. And dried apricots are easy to store and take with you.

What to do: Eat seven or eight dried apricot halves as soon as you notice the symptoms of hypoglycemia, such as fatigue, dizziness, sweating and irritability.

Also helpful: Anything sugary, including a small amount of jelly beans. When your blood sugar is "crashing," you need sugar immediately. Toby Smithson, RD, LDN, a nutritionist who has had diabetes for 40 years, always carries jelly beans. They're even mentioned on the American Diabetes Association website.

Other sources of fast-acting sugars include honey and fruit juices.

Blood Sugar Tip: Eat This, Then That

Study titled "Food Order Has a Significant Impact on Postprandial Glucose and Insulin Levels" by researchers at Weill Cornell Medical College, New York City, published in *Diabetes Care*.

If your blood sugar sometimes runs a little high—and most definitely if you have prediabetes or diabetes—you'll get lots of advice about what to eat but rarely what to eat first in a meal. But the order of what you eat can make a big difference in your blood sugar response.

In a small pilot study of overweight people with type 2 diabetes, on days when they ate carbs at lunch first (ciabatta bread, orange juice), followed 15 minutes later by the foods rich in protein plus some fat (grilled chicken breast, salad with low-fat dressing, steamed broccoli with butter), their blood sugar levels were more than one-third higher 60 minutes later—compared with days on which they reversed the order and ate the protein-rich dish first. Insulin levels were higher, too.

It makes the common practice of munching from the bread basket before your main dish arrives particularly suspect! Instead, whether you're at home or eating out, try starting your meal with something that's high in protein, with some good fats, and perhaps even fiber-rich veggies—for example, veggies and hummus, peanut butter and celery or chilled shrimp with cocktail sauce—before you eat any carb-rich food. What you eat still matters, of course, but eating foods in the right order might help keep your blood sugar levels from spiking after a meal. It also helps if you're a little hungry before you eat.

For Better Blood Sugar, You Can't Beat Beets

Christopher Bell, PhD, department of health and exercise science, Colorado State University, Fort Collins, and coauthor of the research article "Concurrent Beet Juice and Carbohydrate Ingestion: Influence on Glucose Tolerance in Obese and Nonobese Adults," published in *Journal of Nutrition and Metabolism.* "10 Best Juicing Recipes for Diabetics," iFocusHealth.com.

If your blood sugar is too high and you're fighting the battle of the bulge, there's an easy way to enhance your insulin sensitivity and better regulate your blood sugar.

Drink a tall cool glass of beet juice before a meal.

Background: The idea that drinking beet juice has a positive effect on general health is hardly new. Beet juice is rich in dietary nitrate, which the body uses to make nitric oxide, a compound that helps widen blood vessels, improving circulation. Drinking beetroot juice has been shown to reduce blood pressure, improve blood flow to the brain, improve athletic performance and even prevent altitude sickness. Improving circulation also helps the body deliver glucose to the tissues more efficiently so that the body needs to produce less insulin to metabolize food and control blood sugar. But obese people tend to have low nitric oxide levels. Could beets help boost their nitric oxide and improve their insulin sensitivity? To find out, researchers gave people beet juice and a large amount of sugar to digest. It's a way to simulate the effects of a meal in a lab.

Study: Twelve nonobese men and women and 10 obese men and women took part. Being obese is a significant risk factor for developing diabetes, although none of the participants actually had diabetes. They all were asked to not eat any nitrate-rich foods such as beets or greens the day before. They were also asked to not brush their teeth, floss or use mouthwash for 18 hours before the test. On the day of the study, they each drank a 17-ounce glass of beet juice and then were given a large amount of glucose sugar to consume.

On another day, they rinsed with mouthwash—which prevents the body from turning beet's nitrates into nitric oxide—before consuming the beet juice and sugar. It may seem odd to study this—after all, who rinses with mouthwash before a meal? But the researchers had a reason. They knew that the healthful bacteria in the mouth are needed to convert beet's nitrates into nitrites, the first step for the body to make nitric oxide. When you kill the bacteria in your mouth with mouthwash, they aren't around to do the necessary work.

Result: For the obese beet-juice drinkers, insulin resistance was improved and blood sugar didn't go up as much in the 60 to 90 minutes after consuming the sugar—compared to when they rinsed with mouthwash first. Their insulin resistance and blood sugar still were slightly higher than in their nonobese counterparts—but it was a big improvement for them. That's a key benefit, since elevated insulin resistance plus high blood sugar, over time, increase the risk of developing type 2 diabetes. For the obese, who likely started with low nitric oxide levels, drinking beet juice apparently boosted nitric oxide levels high enough to help them better metabolize sugar.

But the beet juice didn't have the same effect on participants who weren't obese—their insulin sensitivity and blood sugar response to eating sugar was normal when they drank beet juice and when they negated the benefits of beet juice by rinsing with mouthwash. Why? One probable reason is that their nitric oxide levels were already sufficient to help their bodies metabolize sugar, so boosting it a little extra with beet juice didn't have any practical effect.

Bottom line: Obese adults at risk of developing insulin resistance may benefit from adding healthful nitrate-rich foods—including a glass of beet juice—to their meals.

What about the sugar naturally contained in beet juice itself? It's true that there's a lot of sugar in beets—and even more in beet juice. But evidence suggests that the physiological benefits outweigh the sugar—just make sure you skip less healthy sources of sugar such as soda, candy and other sweets. You can also experiment with other nitrate-rich foods, such as spinach.

Try this nitrate-rich homemade beet/apple/celery/spinach juice at breakfast: The night before, cut up one medium-sized beet into cubes and freeze it. The next morning, put the cubes in your juicer along with one sliced and cored apple, two chopped celery stalks, one-half cup of spinach and the juice of one small lemon. Like your beets at lunch or dinner instead? Nothing beats roasted beets!

Caution: Before consuming beet juice regularly, ask your doctor whether there's any reason you should avoid or limit foods such as beets, beet juice and spinach. These foods may not be safe for people who are at risk for kidney stones or who are taking certain medications for heart conditions or erectile dysfunction.

Real Mexican Food Fights Diabetes

Margarita Santiago-Torres, PhD, assistant professor, department of internal medicine, University of New Mexico Comprehensive Cancer Center, Albuquerque, and lead author of study titled, "Metabolic responses to a traditional Mexican diet compared with a commonly consumed US diet in women of Mexican descent: a randomized crossover feeding trial," published in *The American Journal of Clinical Nutrition*.

I t's hard to imagine that Mexican food is good for preventing diabetes, let alone protecting you from cancer. Just think about the common gut-busting fare at a typical Mexican restaurant—"loaded" nachos, bottomless bowls of fried tortilla chips, white-flour–based burritos the size of a loaf pan overstuffed with meat and cheese and sour cream. You might get beans…probably fried in fat!

But here's a secret: That's not really Mexican food. The truth is, it's much closer to the typical American diet—one that's high in calories, refined grains, large amounts of meat, with a mere smattering of fresh vegetables and fruit. Real Mexican food, on the other hand, is just as delicious (or more so) and includes plenty of vegetables, legumes, whole grains and fruits plus modest amounts of meat, milk and Mexican cheeses—and is a whole lot healthier. Eating this way may help to prevent diabetes—and it's a healthy way to eat if you already have diabetes.

In the latest research, eating real Mexican food helped healthy women reduce insulin resistance—a key risk factor for developing type 2 diabetes—in just a few weeks.

The Mexican Experiment

At the Fred Hutchinson Cancer Research Center in Seattle, researchers were concerned that women of Mexican descent who adopt an American diet have disproportionately high rates of obesity and diabetes compared to individuals of Mexican descent who keep their more traditional Mexican diets. So they tried an experiment—what if these women went back to eating their traditional Mexican fare?

They recruited 53 healthy women. About half were normal weight and half overweight or obese. None had high blood sugar, diabe-

Yogurt…Not Butter!

When it comes to diabetes risk, food choice is crucial. In a four-year study of nearly 3,500 middle-aged and older men and women at high cardiovascular risk, those who ate an additional three pats of butter a day more than doubled their risk for type 2 diabetes, and each ounce of cheese increased risk by about one-third.

However: Whole milk didn't budge the needle, and each daily 4.5-ounce serving of full-fat yogurt (compared with no yogurt) cut risk by 35%.

What to do: Favor plant-based sources of fat, such as olive oil and nuts, over butter and cheese. Whole milk is fine, and full-fat yogurt is healthy.

Marta Guasch-Ferré, PhD, research fellow, department of nutrition, Harvard T.H. Chan School of Public Health, Boston.

tes, or any other serious health problem. The women were divided into two groups. For 24 days, one group ate a traditional Mexican diet, and the other ate typical American foods and beverages. Both diets were similar in calories and macronutrients (protein, carbohydrates and total fat), and they weren't designed to lead to weight loss. All the meals were prepared for the women. After the initial phase, the women switched diets so that those eating American ate traditional Mexican and vice-versa.

Results: When the women ate traditional Mexican food, their bodies became more sensitive to insulin, so they needed less insulin to digest their meals. That's significant because elevated levels of insulin increase the risk of developing diabetes. *Specifics...*

•**A marker of insulin resistance went down 15% in women eating traditional Mexican food.**

•**Insulin levels went down 14%.**

•**An insulin-related growth factor, which is linked to increased cancer risk, went down 4%.**

Like any study, this one has its limits. It included only women, and only women of Mexican descent at that, so how women and men of other ethnic backgrounds would respond to healthy Mexican food isn't scientifically established. Nor does it mean that the diets that most people eat in Mexico today are healthy—the truth is, there's lots of unhealthful food served in Mexico these days, and rates of obesity and diabetes are sky high on both sides of the border.

But going back to the old food ways might be a solution in Mexico and in the US. Other research has confirmed, for example, that the traditional Mexican dietary pattern is associated with reduced risk of chronic disease in observational studies.

The really good part: If you've never tried real, traditional Mexican food, and you give it a go, you might find that you love it. Here's how to put it to use in your kitchen—and when you go out to Mexican restaurants.

How to Eat Healthy the Mexican Way

What makes traditional Mexican cuisine so much healthier than the typical American diet? Well, first, let's admit what most Americans tend to eat the most of—meat (including processed meat)...mounds of cheese...other processed foods...fried foods...refined carbs...and lots of sugar, including sugar-sweetened beverages.

In contrast, the traditional Mexican meals served in the study featured corn-based dishes cooked with chilies, garlic, onions and herbs, beans, squash, citrus fruits and rice. There was full-fat dairy and cheese, too—yay—but not the same dairy or the same cheese that most Americans eat. (More on that below.)

Margarita Santiago-Torres, PhD, an assistant professor in the department of internal medicine at the University of New Mexico Comprehensive Cancer Center in Albuquerque and one of the study authors, made some interesting distinctions...

•**Real tortillas.** In authentic Mexican cooking, there's no such thing as a "flour tortilla," which is considered a refined grain product and is an American invention. Traditional Mexican tortillas are made only from whole corn, which is high in fiber and offers vegetable protein. And although corn tortillas figure prominently in Mexican cuisine, chips made by frying them do not.

•**Less animal protein.** Most of the protein in traditional Mexican cuisine comes from vegetable sources such as beans and other legumes. The role of meat in a typical meal is minimal. Although meats are incorporated into many meals, they are often in smaller portions in dishes such as pozole (a corn-based soup often made with chicken or pork) and mixed dishes such as tamales. (In the study, while total protein was the same for both diets, the amount from vegetable sources was much higher in the Mexican diet...40 grams a day versus 26 grams).

•**Fiber from food, not from a bottle.** The corn and beans and other legumes that figure so prominently in traditional Mexican dishes are rich in dietary fiber, which is not only important for digestion and helps manage blood sugar but also lets you feel full longer so you're less likely to overeat. In the study, daily fiber on the traditional Mexican diet was 36 grams—on the American diet, it was 15 grams. For overall nutritive value, these naturally healthful sources of fiber beat out the American version—fiber pills or supplemental fiber powder from a can—by a mile.

•**More fresh produce, less processed food.** The proportions of fruits and vegetables are higher in a traditional Mexican diet than in an American one. And you won't find much in the way of canned or processed foods—which tend to be high in sugar and sodium.

Traditional Mexican food does include some elements that are controversial. A common cooking fat is lard—pig fat—which is high in saturated fat. However, there is also controversy about whether saturated fat actually contributes to heart disease—and there's no reason you couldn't substitute a preferred fat for lard in your cooking if you wished.

The Mexican fare also featured full-fat milk, which has more fat and saturated fat than the low-fat or skim milk that so many Americans choose—but here again, there is growing evidence that full-fat milk may actually be beneficial in terms of diabetes prevention. And the cheeses in traditional Mexican cooking, such as queso blanco and queso fresco, tend to be lower in calories and fat than, say, a typical cheddar. How these dietary elements figure into the healthfulness of Mexican food isn't yet known.

But the big picture is known. Like the Mediterranean diet, the traditional Mexican dietary pattern is a healthy model. If you follow it, you'll be eating fewer refined grains, less sugar and sodium, more fiber and more vegetable protein and fresh produce. When you cook at home, consider trying some traditional Mexican dishes.

As for eating out, the good news is that many new Mexican restaurants, both formal and casual, are incorporating Mexican dishes that are more authentic on their menus. At the very least, suggests Dr. Santiago-Torres, the next time you go out for Mexican food, skip the chips, ask for corn tortillas instead of flour, go for black beans, enjoy plenty of salsa—and take a look to see if they have pozole on the menu.

CHAPTER 9

Foods That Fight Stress and Depression

Nature's Stress Fighters

Maria Noël Groves, RH, a clinical herbalist and founder of Wintergreen Botanicals Herbal Clinic & Education Center in Allenstown, New Hampshire. She is registered with the American Herbalists Guild and is certified by the Southwest School of Botanical Medicine. She is the author of *Body into Balance: An Herbal Guide to Holistic Self-Care.* WintergreenBotanicals.com

In today's always-on-the-go, connected-to-everyone world, many of us feel constantly stimulated. No wonder up to 90% of all doctor visits are prompted by stress-related complaints, such as fatigue, pain, high blood pressure and cardiovascular disease.

Of course, a doctor visit usually means another prescription. It's not surprising that sedatives, antidepressants and antianxiety drugs are among the best-selling drugs in the US. While these potent pharmaceuticals may temporarily improve mood and other stress-related symptoms, they're not a permanent fix and often come with side effects.

The best way to deal with stress is with some basic—but critical—lifestyle changes, such as getting regular exercise, eating a healthier diet and maintaining a stress-reducing practice, such as meditation.

To augment those healthy habits, you can often use herbal medicines to help your body (and brain) cope with stress-related symptoms.*

For stress-related disorders, so-called adaptogenic herbs work well. Also known as stress modulators, these herbs can create balance when your body's

*Before trying herbal therapy, consult your pharmacist or seek a naturopathic doctor or clinical herbalist's assistance, especially if you take prescription medications or have a chronic medical condition.

stress-related hormones are too high or too low. The herbs aren't always a substitute for prescription drugs but may help you avoid them.

The following herbs can be taken singly or in combination. If you're combining herbs, be sure to keep their individual properties in mind as they can lessen each other's effects or work in synergy. While you can safely combine most adaptogenic herbs, be aware of what you're eating and drinking. Coffee, for example, can negate the calming effects of many herbs.

Options for herbal therapy: You can take the herbs below as a tea, tincture or capsule. Follow the recommended doses listed on the product labels.

Best Stress-Fighting Herbs

1. Ashwagandha. This nutty-tasting herb gives a mild energy boost. Paradoxically, it can also improve sleepiness at bedtime.

A study in the *Indian Journal of Psychological Medicine* found that people who took ashwagandha for 60 days had levels of cortisol (one of the main stress hormones) that were nearly 28% lower than those who took a placebo. The herb also gives a mild boost to thyroid function.

Caution: Ashwagandha is in the nightshade family. Try a small amount at first if you react to nightshades such as tomatoes and potatoes. If you have hyperthyroid disease or are on thyroid medication, consult your physician before taking ashwagandha.

2. Schizandra. It's a "mid-range" adaptogen that both calms and energizes, depending on what your body needs. It can help people with stress-related insomnia. It's also good for boosting vitality, mood and libido, and is one of the best herbs for stimulating digestion and improving liver detoxification.

Caution: Schizandra occasionally aggravates an active ulcer or gastroesophageal reflux disease (GERD).

Herbs for Anxiety

If you mainly suffer from anxiety or stress-related "nerves," try one of the calming adaptogens...

3. Holy basil. This herb contains eugenol and other aromatic compounds that give it a pleasant odor—and that appear to reduce stress and improve mental clarity.

Studies suggest that holy basil reduces the stress hormone cortisol. In addition, it's often used for reducing anxiety and grief.

You can take this herb as needed or on a long-term basis. I particularly love it as tea and grow it in my garden.

How to try it: Steep one teaspoon to one tablespoon of dried holy basil (or a handful of the fresh herb) in eight ounces of water for 15 minutes. Drink one to three times daily.

4. Gotu kola. There is some evidence that this herb improves brain circulation and mental functions, while also reducing anxiety. The effects of gotu kola are subtle, making it ideal for long-term emotional balance.

You may not notice significant improvements for two to three months, and you can take it for a year or more. You can also safely combine it with other adaptogens, such as holy basil or ashwagandha, if you feel you need more potent (and faster) effects.

Note: Combination stress formulas are readily available on the market and can often be helpful. Take a look at the ingredients and consider each herb's individual benefits and potential side effects. Pick a formula that makes sense for your needs, and listen to your body.

Using these herbs: Most of the herbal adaptogens listed above will have some effect within one to three days, but with regular use, the effects tend to get more pronounced over the course of several weeks. If you don't notice improvement after two months, try one of the other herbs. Side effects, if any, will usually occur within the first day or two.

While you could take any of these herbs as needed—for example, a cup of holy basil tea on a stressful day—they work better when taken regularly for several months to a year. They're generally not dangerous to take on an ongoing basis, but most people find that they don't need them after a while.

Shopping for Herbs

You can find good-quality herbs at your local herb shop or natural-food store. Seek organic herbs whenever possible—they are grown without synthetic chemicals and more likely to be good quality. Some of my favorite brands for capsules and tinctures include Gaia Herbs, Herb Pharm, Oregon's Wild Harvest and MegaFood.

Online sources for dried herbs include Zack Woods Herb Farm (Zack WoodsHerbs.com)…and Mountain Rose Herbs (MountainRoseHerbs.com).

The 10 Very Best Foods to Prevent Depression (and Build a Healthier Brain)

Drew Ramsey, MD, psychiatrist, Columbia University Medical Center, and assistant professor, Columbia University College of Physicians and Surgeons, both in New York City. His latest book is *Eat Complete*. DrewRamseyMD.com

Here's a startling statistic—studies show that people who consume a healthy diet are 40% to 50% less likely to develop depression.

What are the absolutely best nutrients—and most nutrient-packed foods—to protect your brain from depression and other ailments?

What protects mood also protects against dementia and other brain-related conditions. The brain is the biggest asset we have, so we should be selecting foods that specifically nourish the brain.

Here's how to build the healthiest brain possible—starting in your kitchen.

Nutrients Brains Need Most

These key nutrients as the most important...

•**Long-chain omega-3 fatty acids.** There are two major ones. Docosahexaenoic acid (DHA) creates hormones called "neuroprotectins and resolvins" that combat brain inflammation, which is implicated in the development of depression (as well as dementia). Eicosapentaenoic acid (EPA) protects the cardiovascular system, important for a healthy brain.

•**Zinc.** This mineral plays a major role in the development of new brain cells and can boost the efficacy of antidepressant medications.

•**Folate.** Also known as vitamin B-9, folate is needed for good moods and a healthy brain. It helps produce defensin-1, a molecule that protects the brain and increases the concentration of acetylcholine, a neurotransmitter that's crucial to memory and cognition.

•**Iron.** This essential element is a crucial cofactor in the synthesis of mood-regulating neurotransmitters including dopamine and serotonin.

•**Magnesium.** This mineral is required to keep myelin—the insulation of brain cells—healthy. It also increases brain-derived neurotrophic factor (BDNF), which promotes the growth of new neurons and healthy connections among brain cells. A deficiency in magnesium can lead to depression, anxiety, symptoms of ADHD, insomnia and fatigue.

●**Vitamin B-12.** This vitamin, which often is deficient as we age, helps makes neurotransmitters that are key to mood and memory.

●**Vitamin E.** This potent antioxidant vitamin protects polyunsaturated fatty acids in the brain—including DHA. Vitamin E–rich foods, but not supplements, are linked to the prevention of clinical depression as well as slower progression of Alzheimer's disease. One reason may be that most supplements contain only alpha-tocopherol, while other vitamin E compounds, particularly tocotrienols, play important roles in brain function.

●**Dietary fiber.** A high-fiber diet supports healthy gut bacteria (the gut "microbiome"), which growing evidence suggests is key for mental health.

Boosting Your Mood at the Supermarket

The best brain foods are mostly plant-based, but seafood, wild game and even some organ meats make the top of the list, too…

●**Leafy greens such as kale, mustard greens and collard greens**
●**Bell peppers such as red, green and orange**
●**Cruciferous vegetables such as cauliflower, broccoli and cabbage**
●**Berries such as strawberries, raspberries and blueberries**
●**Nuts such as pecans, walnuts, almonds and cashews**
●**Bivalves such as oysters, clams and mussels**
●**Crustaceans such as crab, lobster and shrimp**
●**Fish such as sardines, salmon and fish roe**
●**Organ meats such as liver, poultry giblets and heart**
●**Game and wild meat such as bison, elk and duck**

Eating these nutrient-dense foods is likely to help prevent and treat mental illness. When someone with depression is treated, the real goal is to prevent that person from ever getting depressed again.

Everyday Brain Foods

Not into eating beef heart? Having a little trouble stocking up on elk? When it comes to meat, wild game may not be widely available, but grass-fed beef, which is higher in omega-3 fatty acids than conventionally raised beef, is stocked in most supermarkets—and may be independently associated with protection from depression.

Other foods that didn't make it to the top of the Brain Food Scale but that still are very good for the brain include eggs (iron, zinc), beans (fiber, magnesium, iron) and fruits and vegetables of all colors (fiber, antioxidants). Plus, small quantities of dark chocolate, which gives you a little dopamine rush. Dopamine, he explains, is a neurotransmitter that provides a feeling of reward.

Need an Energy Boost? Best Foods...

Lisa R. Young, PhD, RD, a nutritionist in private practice and an adjunct professor in the department of nutrition and food studies at New York University in New York City. She is the author of *The Portion Teller Plan: The No-Diet Reality Guide to Eating, Cheating, and Losing Weight Permanently.*

Hitting a wall at 3 pm—even though you had a full night's sleep? Your first instinct may be to reach for a cup o' joe or a sugary treat just to keep you going.

Boost Your Mood Naturally

Too-low levels of the powerful neurotransmitter serotonin have been linked to depression, anxiety, irritability and mental decline.

Natural ways to raise serotonin levels: Vigorous aerobic exercise...20 minutes a day of peaceful meditation...learning to replace negative thoughts and reactions with more positive ones...exposure to sunlight or to lamps that mimic its effects...consuming probiotic foods such as pickles, sauerkraut, kefir and yogurt with active cultures...adding the spice turmeric to food...eating foods high in omega-3 fatty acids, such as cold-water fish including halibut, herring and salmon as well as flaxseed oil and walnuts.

Massachusetts General Hospital's publication *Mind, Mood & Memory.*

Why this is a mistake: It's common for our blood sugar levels to drop in the late afternoon, making us feel tired and hungry. But the mind-buzzing, heart-racing effects of so-called quick fixes soon lead to a crash-and-burn, putting us right back where we started.

What Works Better

Once you accept that quick fixes are really nothing more than "fool's gold," you can embrace the true source of sustained vitality—energy-producing real foods.

What you need to know: Often it is not a single ingredient itself that invigorates but how that powerhouse is combined with flavorful and nutritionally satisfying add-ons.

Rule of thumb: The best foods for natural all-day vibrancy typically balance a complex carbohydrate with a healthy fat and a punch of protein—a combination that takes longer to digest and stabilizes blood sugar levels for hours.

For advice on the best foods to eat for all-day energy, we spoke with leading nutritionist Lisa Young, PhD, RD, CDN, to learn about her top choices for maintaining day-long vim and vigor...

Avocado

Avocado contains heart-healthy monounsaturated fat and provides nearly 20 vitamins and minerals.

My favorite way to eat avocado: Sliced or smashed on whole-grain toast. In addition to being a perfect base for creamy avocado, whole-grain toast boasts its own benefits and makes for a great energy-boosting combo—it fills you up with fiber and is low in saturated fat.

Canned Salmon

What's easier than peeling back the lid on a ready-to-serve portion of this versatile, tasty fish? Especially when two ounces of canned salmon contain just 90 calories and only 1 g of saturated fat in a convenient protein source.

Note: To reduce possible toxins, I recommend wild salmon sold in a BPA-free can.

My favorite way to eat canned salmon: On salad greens topped with heart-smart olive oil and a side of polenta. Cornmeal-based polenta, which is loaded with complex carbs to keep blood sugar levels stable for hours, even comes in ready-made refrigerated tubes. You can cook up a slice or two in just minutes on the stove or in the oven!

Farmer's Cheese

Protein-packed foods such as farmer's cheese—born from farmers' efforts to use milk left over after cream is skimmed for butter—can help you stay on top of your game. Two tablespoons of farmer's cheese offer 4 g of protein with only 2.5 g of fat and 40 calories.

My favorite way to eat farmer's cheese: On Ezekiel 4:9 bread with cinnamon and/or fresh walnuts on top. You can spread farmer's cheese, with its ricotta-like texture, on Ezekiel bread—itself an efficient protein source as well as a unique blend of six grains and legumes. A dash of cinnamon not only adds the yin-yang of sweet and savory, but also helps control blood sugar levels. A few diced walnuts provide satisfying crunch and omega-3 fats that promote cardiovascular health.

Quinoa

Quinoa (pronounced "keen-wah") contains iron, B vitamins, magnesium, calcium, potassium and other nutrients, boasting zero saturated or trans fats. Even better, it takes only about 15 minutes to prepare.

My favorite way to eat quinoa: With chopped veggies and garnished with chickpeas. By topping with chickpeas, you'll boost the overall protein, vitamin and mineral content—and stay fuller longer. Or you can try a quinoa-based hot cereal.

Sorghum

Sorghum, a substantial source of protein and dietary fiber, is a versatile, gluten-free grain that keeps your belly full and your energy levels high.

My favorite way to eat sorghum: In a tomato and red pepper slaw.

To prepare: After simmering and draining your desired amount of sorghum, add some color by folding in a julienned slaw of tomatoes and red peppers.

Tomatoes, with their energy-boosting carbs and fiber, are also a major source of the anticancer nutrient lycopene...while red peppers aid in the absorption of iron from food, which boosts energy by promoting optimal blood oxygen levels.

Six Foods Proven to Make You Happy

Tonia Reinhard, MS, RD, a registered dietitian and professor at Wayne State University in Detroit. She is the program director for the Coordinated Program in Dietetics, course director of clinical nutrition at Wayne State University School of Medicine and past president of the Michigan Academy of Nutrition and Dietetics. She is author of *Superfoods: The Healthiest Foods on the Planet* and *SuperJuicing: More Than 100 Nutritious Vegetable & Fruit Recipes.*

You can eat your way to a better mood! Certain foods and beverages have been proven to provide the raw materials that you need to feel sharper, more relaxed and just plain happier. *Best choices...*

Happy Food #1: Chocolate

Chocolate can make you feel good—to such an extent that 52% of women would choose chocolate over sex, according to one survey.

Chocolate contains chemical compounds known as polyphenols, which interact with neurotransmitters in the brain and reduce anxiety. An Australian study found that men and women who consumed the most chocolate polyphenols (in the form of a beverage) felt calmer and more content than those who consumed a placebo drink.

Chocolate also boosts serotonin, the same neurotransmitter affected by antidepressant medications. It triggers the release of dopamine and stimulates the "pleasure" parts of the brain.

Then there's the sensual side of chocolate—the intensity of the flavor and the melting sensation as it dissolves in your mouth. The satisfaction that people get from chocolate could be as helpful for happiness as its chemical composition.

Recommended amount: Aim for one ounce of dark chocolate a day. Most studies used dark chocolate with 70% cacao or more.

Happy Food #2: Fish

Fish has been called "brain food" because our brains have a high concentration of omega-3 fatty acids—and so does fish. These fatty acids have been linked to memory and other cognitive functions. In countries where people eat a lot of fish, depression occurs less often than in countries (such as the US) where people eat less.

The omega-3s in fish accumulate in the brain and increase "membrane fluidity," the ability of brain-cell membranes to absorb nutrients and transmit chemical signals.

A study in *Archives of General Psychiatry* looked at patients diagnosed with depression who hadn't responded well to antidepressants. Those who were given 1,000 mg of EPA (a type of omega-3 fatty acid) daily for three months had significant improvements, including less anxiety and better sleep.

Recommended amount: Try to have at least two or three fish meals a week. Cold-water fish—such as sardines, mackerel and salmon—have the highest levels of omega-3s. Or choose a supplement with 1,000 mg of EPA and DHA (another omega-3 fatty acid) in total.

Happy Food #3: Dark Green Veggies

Dark green vegetables such as spinach, asparagus, broccoli and Brussels sprouts are loaded with folate, a B-complex vitamin that plays a key role in regulating mood. A Harvard study found that up to 38% of adults with depression had low or borderline levels of folate. Boosting the folate levels of depressed patients improved their mood.

Dark green vegetables are particularly good, but all vegetables and fruits boost mood. Researchers asked 281 people to note their moods on different days. On the days when the participants consumed the most vegetables and fruits, they reported feeling happier and more energetic. Folate certainly plays a role, but self-satisfaction may have something to do with it as well. People feel good when they eat right and take care of themselves.

Recommended amount: The minimum you should have is five servings of vegetables and fruits a day.

Bonus: Middle-aged men who had 10 servings a day showed reduced blood pressure.

Happy Food #4: Beans (Including Soybeans)

Beans are rich in tryptophan, an essential amino acid that is used by the body to produce serotonin, the neurotransmitter that affects feelings of calmness and relaxation.

Beans also are loaded with folate. Folate, as mentioned in the veggies section, plays a key role in regulating mood.

In addition, beans contain manganese, a trace element that helps prevent mood swings due to low blood sugar.

Recommended amount: For people not used to eating beans, start with one-quarter cup five days a week. Build up to one-half cup daily. This progression will help prevent gastrointestinal symptoms such as flatulence.

Happy Food #5: Nuts

Nuts are high in magnesium, a trace mineral involved in more than 300 processes in the body. People who don't get enough magnesium feel irritable, fatigued and susceptible to stress.

The elderly are more likely than young adults to be low in magnesium—because they don't eat enough magnesium-rich foods and/or because they tend to excrete more magnesium in their urine.

Also, many health problems can accelerate the depletion of magnesium from the body.

Examples: Gastrointestinal disorders (or bariatric surgery), kidney disease and sometimes diabetes.

Recommended amount: Aim for one ounce of nuts a day. Good choices include almonds, walnuts, cashews, hazelnuts and peanuts (the latter is technically a legume). If you don't like nuts, other high-magnesium foods include spinach, pumpkin seeds, fish, beans, whole grains and dairy.

Happy Food #6: Coffee

The caffeine in coffee, tea and other caffeinated beverages is a very beneficial compound. One study found that people with mild cognitive impairment were less likely to develop full-fledged Alzheimer's disease when they had the caffeine equivalent of about three cups of coffee a day.

Caffeine can temporarily improve your memory and performance on tests. It enhances coordination and other parameters of physical performance. When you feel energized, you feel happier. Also, people who feel good from caffeine may be more likely to engage in other happiness-promoting behaviors, such as seeing friends and exercising.

Recommended amount: The challenge is finding the "sweet spot"—just enough caffeine to boost mood but not so much that you get the shakes or start feeling anxious. For those who aren't overly sensitive to caffeine, one to three daily cups of coffee or tea are about right.

What Not to Eat

Some people turn to food or drink for comfort when they're feeling down. Here's what not to eat or drink when you've got the blues....

Alcohol: Alcohol is a depressant of the central nervous system. When you initially consume alcohol, it produces a euphoric effect and you become more animated and less inhibited. But as you continue drinking and more alcohol crosses the blood-brain barrier, the depressant effect predominates.

Baked goods: When you eat high-sugar, high-fat carbs such as cookies, pastries and donuts, you tend to want more of them. The food gives you a temporary "good feeling," but the excess food intake that typically results causes drowsiness and often self-loathing.

The Fruit That Fights Insomnia

David Grotto, RD, LDN, a registered dietitian and founder and president of Nutrition Housecall, LLC, a Chicago-based nutrition consulting firm. He is author of *The Best Things You Can Eat.* DavidGrotto.com

Don't depend on warm milk when you can't get to sleep. It does produce some of the relaxing hormone serotonin, but it isn't particularly helpful by itself.

Best food: Tart cherries. They're among the richest food sources of melatonin, the same sleep-inducing hormone that is produced by the pineal gland in the brain. The body's production of melatonin declines with age, which is part of the reason that older adults often have trouble sleeping. A study in *Journal of Clinical Endocrinology & Metabolism* found that small doses of melatonin—about 0.3 milligrams (mg)—helped insomniacs get a better night's sleep. One cup of tart-cherry juice or about one-eighth of a cup of dried tart cherries contains roughly the same amount. Sweet cherries also contain melatonin but not as much.

What to do: Eat tart cherries or drink one cup of juice about an hour before bedtime. The juice is very tart—you might want to mix in a little apple or pineapple juice.

Superfoods for Digestive Health and Bladder Control

Delicious Homemade Drinks for Better Digestion

Meg Thompson, ND, a naturopath and holistic nutritionist in private practice specializing in digestive, women's and children's health in Melbourne, Australia. She is the author of *Superfoods for Life: Cultured and Fermented Beverages* and writes a blog on the benefits of a diet diverse in fresh and whole foods, including numerous recipes, at MyWholeFoodRomance.com.

Oh, our poor digestive tracts! One of the biggest threats is antibiotics, which kill off both harmful bacteria and beneficial bacteria that are needed to keep our digestive systems running smoothly.

But there are additional threats, too, such as drinking too much alcohol or coffee...long-term use of medications such as nonsteroidal anti-inflammatory drugs (NSAIDs) and corticosteroids...eating a poor diet...and living with chronic stress.

The result is often bloating, intestinal gas, constipation, diarrhea, irritable bowel syndrome and other conditions.

Great-tasting way to protect your gut: Drinking kefir, which is bursting with a wide variety of beneficial bacteria—it improves digestion and boosts immunity.

What Is Kefir?

Kefir is a thick, creamy, drinkable liquid that is similar to yogurt, but it tastes more tart and has more beneficial bacteria, including a variety of Lactobacillus species and beneficial yeasts. When kefir is consumed, it coats the digestive tract, giving beneficial bacteria a place to settle and colonize. To build up and maintain your levels of beneficial bacteria, consider drinking one cup of kefir daily.

You can make your own "basic milk kefir" for the delicious, health-promoting recipes here…or use plain store-bought kefir.

BASIC MILK KEFIR

This drink can be consumed on its own, or it can be added to smoothies, dressings and desserts.

1 cup refrigerated organic cow's milk

1½ teaspoons milk kefir grains*

1 sterilized glass jar,** no lid (about 1¼ cups or larger)

1 sterilized glass jar with lid (about 1¼ cups)

1 small piece of cheesecloth or paper towel

1 rubber band

1 fine-mesh strainer

Pour milk into a glass jar with no lid and add kefir grains. Secure the cheese-cloth on top of the jar with a rubber band and store at room temperature for 12 to 24 hours. Depending on the temperature in your home and how sour you like your kefir (the longer it ferments, the more sour it will taste), fermentation can take up to 48 hours. Strain the kefir through the mesh strainer into the second jar, and seal with a lid. It will last in the refrigerator for one week. Transfer remaining kefir grains from the strainer into a new jar to begin a new batch.

Yield: 1 cup. For larger batches, double or triple all ingredients (using larger jars).

ANTIBIOTIC REPAIR KIT SMOOTHIE

Drink this delicious smoothie to replenish the beneficial bacteria while (and after) taking antibiotics.

1 cup basic milk (or store-bought) kefir

1 peeled banana

2 Tablespoons rolled oats (any type)

---

*Kefir grains can be purchased online at CulturesforHealth.com. All fermented and cultured beverages, such as kefir, contain some alcohol, but the percentage is typically only about 0.5%, which is considered "nonalcoholic."

**Sterilize glass jars by placing them in boiling water for five minutes, then let cool before using.

Add all of the ingredients to a blender, and blend on high speed until smooth. Drink immediately.

Yield: 1½ cups.

APPLE PIE KEFIR WITH CRUNCHY GRANOLA TOPPING

This tasty drink is just as comforting and homey as apple pie!

2 Tablespoons rolled oats (any type)

2 Tablespoons unsweetened coconut flakes

2 Tablespoons coarsely chopped, raw, unsalted almonds

1 cup basic milk (or store-bought) kefir

1 apple (preferably organic), cored and coarsely chopped

½ teaspoon ground cinnamon

¼ teaspoon ground nutmeg

¼ teaspoon pure vanilla extract

1 Tablespoon pure maple syrup (optional)

Preheat the oven to 350°F. Place the oats, coconut flakes and almonds on a baking sheet, and bake for 12 minutes or until the coconut just starts to brown a little. Remove from the oven, and allow to cool. Put the kefir, apple, cinnamon, nutmeg, vanilla and maple syrup in a blender, and blend until smooth. Pour into a glass, and top with the topping mix.

Yield: 1½ cups.

Raisins for Reducing Nighttime Bathroom Visits

Joe Graedon, MS, a pharmacologist, and Terry Graedon, PhD, a medical anthropologist. The Graedons are coauthors of *The People's Pharmacy Quick & Handy Home Remedies* and cohosts of *The People's Pharmacy* public radio program. Joe Graedon is an adjunct assistant professor in the division of practice advancement and clinical education at the University of North Carolina Eshelman School of Pharmacy at Chapel Hill, and Terry Graedon is a founding member of Duke University Health System's Patient Advocacy Council, Durham. PeoplesPharmacy.com

Getting out of bed multiple times a night to urinate isn't just annoying, it's actually a proven predictor of mortality. That's because sleep disruption predisposes you to a number of chronic illnesses, such as hypertension and heart disease.

As far as we know, there's no scientific research to support this remedy, but we've heard many times that it works. One woman told us that two spoonfuls of raisins before bed helped her reduce bathroom visits from once every hour or two to about once a night. And another writer claimed that eating 10 raisins three times a day allowed him to stop taking bladder medication!

Important: Never stop taking a prescription medication without consulting your doctor first.

What to do: Try eating a tablespoon of raisins before you brush and floss your teeth at night.

Parsley Eases UTIs

Michael T. Murray, ND, a licensed naturopathic physician based in Paradise Valley, Arizona. Dr. Murray has published more than 30 books, including *Bottom Line's Encyclopedia of Healing Foods*, with coauthor Joseph Pizzorno, ND. DoctorMurray.com

Most people think of parsley as a colorful garnish—pretty to look at, but not much of a food. But around the world, parsley is found in tabbouleh, pesto (with or without basil) and other fragrant dishes... and it's a good green to eat if you get frequent urinary tract infections (UTIs).

About half of all women will eventually get a UTI...men get them, too, but less often. Patients with recurrent UTIs (defined as two separate infections within six months or three within one year) often depend on antibiotics—and resign themselves to the likely side effects of these drugs, such as diarrhea.

How parsley helps: It contains *apigenin*, a compound that acts as a diuretic and also has anti-inflammatory effects. According to a report in the journal *Case Reports in Medicine*, women who combined parsley with other herbal treatments (such as garlic) had an impressive decrease in urinary frequency and other symptoms—by 80%, in one case. Parsley's UTI-fighting effect is presumably because of apigenin's diuretic effect.

> **Quick Food Fix for Constipation**
>
> Eating three dried figs a day can relieve chronic constipation, according to a recent eight-week clinical trial.
>
> *Asian Journal of Clinical Nutrition.*

Another benefit: Reduced risk for cancer. Chlorophyll and other compounds in parsley have anticancer effects—including the ability to help inhibit the cancer-causing effects of fried foods.

Since parsley is so concentrated in nutrition and phytochemicals, just a few sprigs (or about one-quarter cup) consumed whenever possible provides exceptional health benefits. Chopped parsley can be added to salads, sauces, soups and grilled fish.

Four Food (and Drink) Secrets for a Super Liver

Michelle Lai, MD, MPH, an assistant professor of medicine at Harvard Medical School and a hepatologist at Beth Israel Deaconess Medical Center, both in Boston. Dr. Lai is coauthor of *The Liver Healing Diet.* Her research frequently appears in peer-reviewed journals such as *The New England Journal of Medicine* and the *Journal of Hepatology.*

Most people assume that liver disease happens only to people who abuse alcohol. But that is not true.

Surprising facts: More than 30 million US adults suffer from chronic liver disease—and many of these people don't even know that they have it. Liver problems can be caused by a number of conditions such as fatty liver disease (see below) and hepatitis C and hepatitis B. The result can range from mild dysfunction to cirrhosis, liver failure and liver cancer.

An under-recognized problem: A condition called nonalcoholic fatty liver disease (NAFLD). Affecting as many as one in four adults in this country, it is marked by a buildup of extra fat in the liver cells. This can allow a more serious condition to develop that can result in liver scarring and cirrhosis—problems that may lead to liver failure or cancer, requiring a liver transplant.

Keeping Your Liver Healthy

Your liver is one of the hardest-working—and underappreciated—organs in your body. It's responsible for more than 500 critical functions, ranging from digesting and storing nutrients to processing and excreting toxic substances that sneak into your body via food, drink and air. If your liver gets sick, you get sick—it's that simple.

Fortunately, there are simple steps you can take to help protect your liver health. *My advice...*

•**Fight unwanted weight gain.** This is key to liver health. For most people, a crucial part of maintaining a healthy body weight is to cut back on their sugar intake.

Besides promoting system-wide inflammation and weight gain, excessive sugar (typically from sweets, soda, fruit drinks and other flavored beverages) can cause your liver to become fatty and inflamed—thus contributing to NAFLD.

Important: The 2015–2020 edition of the federal *Dietary Guidelines* calls for us to limit our added sugar intake to less than 10% of daily calories—the equivalent of roughly 10 to 15 teaspoons of sugar per day.

Some easy ways to cut back on sugar in your diet: Switch from flavored yogurt to plain Greek yogurt topped with fruit…and substitute unsweetened applesauce for refined white sugar when baking.

•**Drink coffee.** Scientific evidence continues to shore up coffee's protective effect on the liver—perhaps due to its inflammation-fighting properties.

Important recent findings: A March 2015 World Cancer Research Fund study found that each cup of coffee you drink per day reduces your risk for liver cancer by 14%. An analysis of other studies showed that drinking two cups of coffee per day may reduce risk for cirrhosis by 44%.

Helpful: Opt for caffeinated coffee and, if possible, have it black. Sugar, of course, causes inflammation, and decaf java has not been shown in research to have the same liver-friendly benefits.

•**Try wheat germ.** With its mild, nutty taste, wheat germ is an excellent source of vitamin E. Two tablespoons of ready-to-eat wheat germ provide 5.4 mg of vitamin E—about one-third of your daily needs. Why is this vitamin so important? Animal studies suggest that wheat germ can help protect the liver against toxins. While human data is limited, a study of 132,000 Chinese adults found that as vitamin E intake rose, the likelihood of liver cancer dropped.

Wheat germ is also rich in essential fatty acids, potassium and magnesium—all of which help ease oxidative stress on the liver by protecting the body's cells from free radical damage.

Helpful: Sprinkle wheat germ over oatmeal, yogurt or popcorn…or mix it into meatloaf or smoothies. For other good sources of vitamin E, try almonds, spinach, avocado and sunflower seeds.

•**Choose seafood wisely.** Fish is an excellent source of protein, vitamins and minerals and heart-healthy omega-3 fatty acids. However, many types of fish can accumulate heavy metals, such as mercury, lead and cadmium, from the water and the aquatic life they consume. When we eat such fish, we ingest these toxins, which, over time, can cause liver damage.

Self-defense: Select seafood that is less likely to contain heavy metals. For example, you can safely enjoy 12 ounces a week of smaller fish such as anchovies…catfish… flounder…herring…perch…wild salmon… sardines…and trout.

Vinegar for Gut Health
Mice with ulcerative colitis had fewer symptoms when vinegar was added to their drinking water.
Possible reasons: Vinegar may increase levels of beneficial intestinal bacteria, while suppressing pro-inflammatory proteins.
Journal of Agricultural and Food Chemistry.

Caution: Limit your intake of fish that may contain higher levels of heavy metals such as Chilean sea bass…grouper…mackerel…and yellowfin and white albacore tuna to less than 18 ounces per month.

Avoid large fish such as marlin…orange roughy…ahi tuna…and swordfish—these fish usually contain the highest levels of heavy metals.

Helpful: Visit the Natural Resources Defense Council at NRDC.org for a complete list of the safest seafood options.

•**Don't forget water!** Water makes the liver's job easier by helping flush toxins out of the body. It's also a sugar-free substitute for juice, soda, sweetened tea and other sugar-enhanced beverages.

Helpful: Keep a glass of water on your nightstand, and start your morning with it, then continue sipping all day long. To jazz up your water, try adding freshly cut slices of citrus.

Herbs and Foods for Leaky Gut

Jamison Starbuck, ND, a naturopathic physician in family practice and a guest lecturer at the University of Montana, both in Missoula. She is past president of the American Association of Naturopathic Physicians. Dr. Starbuck is a columnist in *Bottom Line Health* newsletter, and hosts "Dr. Starbuck's Health Tips for Kids" on Montana Public Radio. DrJamisonStarbuck.com

I f you've got celiac disease, food allergies or an autoimmune bowel disease, such as Crohn's disease or inflammatory bowel disease, you probably have leaky gut syndrome. Also known as gastrointestinal permeability, leaky gut syndrome is a condition in which microscopic "holes" develop in the lining of the digestive tract as a result of medications, allergies to foods, genetics and other causes. Your digestive tract, or gut, is designed to keep food particles in your intestines and out of your bloodstream. When food is properly digested and broken down, food nutrients pass through the filter of the intestinal wall and into the bloodstream. This is how your body gets the nutrition it needs to survive.

With leaky gut syndrome, your gut wall is like a torn window screen. Insects that are meant to stay outside enter your home. When leaky gut occurs, overly large food molecules pass through these microscopic holes into your bloodstream. To the body, these large molecules are an enemy. The immune system responds protectively and makes defenders known as antibodies. If you have a lot of food-related antibodies, you have food allergies (or a food sensitivity). You'll also have an inflamed bowel and leaky gut syndrome.

One way to heal the symptoms of leaky gut syndrome, which include indigestion, irregular stools, generalized fatigue and inflammation, skin rashes and migraines, is to avoid the foods to which you are allergic. That can help. However, if you don't repair the intestinal wall, you'll continue to suffer with many of the above symptoms and may even become allergic to other foods.

How, then, do you treat the gut wall? *What I recommend…*

•**Eat the right foods.** Sauerkraut is rich in probiotics, which help crowd out pathogens that damage the gut wall. Do not use canned sauerkraut—the probiotics are killed in the heating process that is required for canning. Plant-based oils, such as olive, sunflower and borage, are nourishing to the intestine. Fish, baked or cooked on a grill, can also help heal a leaky gut. It is easy to digest, anti-inflammatory and contains helpful proteins and oils. Just be sure to avoid fried fish and fried foods generally. You may also want to try a probiotic supplement. Follow label instructions.

Caution: People with weakened immune systems (such as those using chemotherapy) should consult their doctors before eating probiotic-rich food or taking a probiotic supplement.

•**Consider these herbs.** My favorite herbs for leaky gut are slippery elm… marshmallow root…and plantain (a medicinal plant not to be confused with the banana-like food). You can use one of these herbs or combine two or more.

To treat leaky gut: You need to take herbal medicine between meals—60 minutes or more after a meal or 30 minutes or more before a meal—to ensure that the herb comes into direct contact with the gut wall.* You can take these herbs in capsules, tea or bulk powders.

Typical daily dose: Three standard-sized capsules two times a day…three cups of tea…or two teaspoons of the bulk-powdered herb. For convenience

*If you use any prescription medication, have a chronic medical condition (such as diabetes) or are pregnant or nursing, consult your doctor before taking any herbs.

and taste, put the powdered herb in a small amount (one-eighth cup or less) of applesauce or oatmeal.

With my patients, treatment usually takes about three months to heal leaky gut. Assuming that one's diet stays healthy, the regimen above can often be discontinued when symptoms subside.

Coca-Cola Cures Bezoars

Dimitrios Kamberoglou, MD, consultant gastroenterologist, gastroenterology division, First Department of Medicine–Propaedeutic, Medical School, Athens University, Laikon Hospital, Greece.

You've surely heard several health warnings concerning soda. Well, it turns out that there is a situation in which soda may be used as medicine. Surprised? This concerns a certain digestive ailment. *Here's the deal...*

You probably assume that the food you eat starts getting digested in your stomach, finishes the digestion process in your intestines and then leaves your body via the "back door." And usually that is what happens. But not always!

Sometimes foods don't get fully digested—and the undigested bits clump together to form a hard chunk that gets stuck in your intestines. This chunk is called a bezoar.

Bezoars can cause nasty symptoms, such as feeling full after eating only a small amount of food, abdominal pain and vomiting. The chunks also can lead to gastric ulcers, intestinal bleeding, intestinal obstruction and even gangrene of the digestive tract. So treatment is definitely warranted—yet treatments can be invasive and costly and they have side effects and risks, as well.

That's why you should know about a new study on an underused treatment that is simple, safe and cheap. This is where (believe it or not) the soda comes in.

Bezoar Basics

People at highest risk for bezoars are those with diabetes or end-stage kidney disease or those who have had gastric surgery. Seniors

Pantry Cure for Heartburn

If you have a bout of heartburn and you've run out of antacids or prefer a safe, natural way to feeling better, take a teaspoon or two of uncooked oatmeal flakes (old-fashioned kind is best), and chew thoroughly before swallowing. Oatmeal absorbs the stomach acid that can cause the burning pain of indigestion.

Joan Wilen and Lydia Wilen are folk-remedy experts based in New York City who have spent decades collecting "cures from the cupboard." They are authors of *Bottom Line's Treasury of Home Remedies & Natural Cures* and *Bottom Line's Household Magic.*

also are at increased risk because aging decreases stomach acid and diminishes chewing efficiency. Use of certain drugs that interfere with digestion can contribute to risk, too. But the fact is that anyone can develop a bezoar.

Of the several different types of bezoars, the most common is a phytobezoar, which is composed of indigestible food fibers, such as cellulose from fruits and vegetables. Not all high-fiber foods are problematic—but particular culprits do include prunes, raisins, persimmons and pineapples...beets, celery, pumpkins and leeks...and sunflower seed husks.

Fizzy Solution

Scientists in Greece combed through 10 years of research done in various countries—24 studies covering 46 patients in total—showing that using Coca-Cola was an effective treatment for phytobezoars.

Most patients either drank the Coke or got it via a nasogastric tube. Different amounts of Coke were used in different studies, and the frequency of the dosages also varied. But typically, patients drank the soda over the course of as little as 24 hours or as long as six weeks. When the Coke was given through a nasogastric tube, it was usually administered over a 12-hour period.

Results: Using Coke alone completely dissolved half the bezoars. For another 40%, Coke was used first to make the bezoar smaller and softer, and then the remaining chunk was either broken up or removed using an endoscopic tool inserted into the stomach.

This is very encouraging news, when you consider the other treatment options for bezoars. Sometimes doctors have patients ingest an enzyme such as papain or cellulase. But papain may increase the risk for gastric ulcer, and cases of small bowel obstruction have occurred after treatment with cellulase. There's also endoscopy and, as a last resort, surgery—both of which are expensive, invasive and carry risks (such as infection).

In comparison, the Coke treatment holds appeal even for people who normally avoid soda like the plague. In fact, 50% of all bezoar patients in the studies who got the Coke therapy were able to avoid all of the other treatments mentioned above—and 90% of them were able to avoid surgery.

Coke Mimics Stomach Acid

Only regular (full-sugar) Coke was used in the studies, but past research has shown that Diet Coke and Coca-Cola Zero are equally effective at breaking down bezoars. That's because all versions are highly acidic and resemble the natural stomach acid that's necessary to properly digest fiber. Also, the fizzy drinks' carbonation may enhance this dissolving effect. The researchers in the Greek study did not think that the caffeine in cola was a factor in combating bezoars.

Are other brands of cola as effective as Coke? They probably would be, but the researchers had no experience with using other brands for this purpose. And there is no data to suggest whether noncola soft drinks (such as Sprite) would be effective against bezoars.

Are you at high risk of developing a bezoar, or have you had one in the past? *Here's a list of prevention strategies...*

- **Chew your food thoroughly.**

- **Drink plenty of water throughout the day to avoid dehydration.**

- **Don't stop eating fruits and veggies** (you need their nutrients!), but avoid persimmons and pineapples because those fruits can cause especially hard bezoars that are difficult to treat.

- **Consider drinking a daily glass or two of cola.** Although this hasn't been studied explicitly, the drink may help prevent bezoars from forming in the first place.

Caveat: Drinking regular Coke, of course, increases your risk for obesity, high blood sugar and other health problems...and though Diet Coke and Coca-Cola Zero have no calories, there are concerns about their artificial sweeteners—so first discuss the benefits and risks with your doctor.

And if you ever do experience possible symptoms of a bezoar? Visit your doctor, who can diagnose the problem with either an imaging test or endoscopic test. Then show this article to your physician—in case he or she isn't aware of this "Coke therapy."

CHAPTER 11

Superfoods for Women's Health

Boost Your Sex Drive Naturally!

Laurie Steelsmith, ND, LAc, a licensed naturopathic physician and acupuncturist with a 20-year private practice in Honolulu. Dr. Steelsmith is coauthor of *Great Sex, Naturally: Every Woman's Guide to Enhancing Her Sexuality Through the Secrets of Natural Medicine.* DrLaurieSteelsmith.com

D iminished libido—little or no sexual desire—is the most common sexual complaint among women. But repeated attempts by the pharmaceutical industry to solve the problem with one or another form of "female Viagra" have failed.

My viewpoint: Reviving a mature woman's sex drive requires addressing multiple factors. *These include...*

• **Balancing hormones**—which play a key role in both physical and mental aspects of arousal—particularly during the hormonal changes of perimenopause and menopause.

• **Treating the pelvic problems of aging,** such as vaginal atrophy and dryness, which can cause painful sex.

Here are natural ways to boost libido that consistently work for the mature women in my medical practice. Choose one or two based on your particular needs. If you still have problems, consult a licensed naturopathic physician.

Hormone Help

Several herbs and herbal combinations can help balance a mature woman's hormones. *Two of my favorites...*

•**Maca.** This powerful Peruvian herb is a good choice for women going through perimenopause or menopause because it is rich in plant sterols that balance and strengthen the entire hormonal system. The herb not only increases sex drive but also improves perimenopausal and menopausal symptoms such as hot flashes, night sweats and insomnia.

Additionally, it supports the adrenal glands, reducing levels of energy-depleting stress hormones.

Typical dose: 1,000 milligrams (mg), twice daily.

•**Two Immortals.** This herbal formula from Traditional Chinese Medicine builds two types of chi, or life-energy—yin (feminine) chi and yang (masculine) chi—thereby boosting a woman's libido, which requires both nurturing (yin) and stimulation (yang).

It also helps to balance hormones and control some symptoms of perimenopause (irregular menstrual bleeding and cramping) and menopause (hot flashes).

Many of my patients take it for six months to a year to rebuild their vitality.

Typical dose: Many companies manufacture the supplement, and dosages vary—follow the dosage recommendation on the label.

Super-Sex Supplements

Two nutritional supplements are particularly effective at stimulating sexuality...

•**L-arginine.** This amino acid works by boosting nitric oxide, a compound that promotes blood flow—including blood flow to your genitals.

A study in *Journal of Sex & Marital Therapy* showed that more than 70% of women who took a supplement containing L-arginine (ArginMax for Women) experienced increased sexual desire, more frequent sex and orgasm, enhanced clitoral stimulation, decreased vaginal dryness and improved overall sexual satisfaction.

Typical dose: 3,000 mg daily.

Caution: Talk to your doctor before you take L-arginine, especially if you have low blood pressure, herpes, gastric ulcer, liver disease or kidney disease.

•**PEA (*phenylethylamine*).** Called the "love supplement," PEA boosts the neurotransmitter dopamine, enhancing feelings of well-being, joy and pleasure.

Typical dose: 60 mg once a day. (Higher doses can cause overstimulation, insomnia or anxiety.)

Caution: Don't take PEA if you're nursing, pregnant or take an MAOI antidepressant medication such as selegiline (Eldepryl).

You also can boost PEA by exercising regularly, eating dark chocolate and taking a blue-green algae called spirulina.

Aphrodisiacs

Two aphrodisiacs are particularly effective for mature women because—by relaxing your body and improving your mood—they slowly and gently boost your libido.

•**Cordyceps.** This mushroom is considered a potent sexual tonic in Traditional Chinese Medicine. It enhances both yin and yang chi, making it an ideal aphrodisiac for women.

Typical dose: 500 mg, twice daily.

What works best: Pills made by a hot-water extraction process that pulls out the herb's most active constituents, such as the cordyceps supplement from JHS Natural Products.

•**Ginkgo biloba.** Often recommended for memory loss because it improves blood supply to the brain, ginkgo also promotes blood flow to the vulva and vagina. Studies show that it may help restore libido in women taking antidepressants, which can destroy sex drive.

Typical dose: 40 mg, three times a day. The label should read, "Standardized extract of 24% ginkgo flavonglycosides (or flavone glycosides)."

Eating Oranges May Cut Women's Stroke Risk

Aedin Cassidy, PhD, professor of diet and health, Norwich Medical School, University of East Anglia, Norwich, United Kingdom.

Researchers studied the health records of 69,622 women, who reported their food intake every four years for 14 years.

Result: Women whose diets contained high levels of flavanones (found in oranges, grapefruit and other citrus fruit) had a 19% lower risk for ischemic stroke (caused by a blood clot) than those who ate the least amount of flavanones.

Theory: Flavanones are thought to improve blood vessel function and have anti-inflammatory qualities.

Caution: Because grapefruit can interact with some medications, speak to your doctor before increasing your intake.

Natural Cures for Women's Vexing Health Problems

Tori Hudson, ND, a naturopathic physician, medical director of A Woman's Time Health Clinic in Portland, Oregon, and program director of the Institute of Women's Health & Integrative Medicine. Dr. Hudson is also an adjunct clinical professor at Bastyr University in Kenmore, Washington, the National College of Naturopathic Medicine in Portland, Oregon, and the Southwest College of Naturopathic Medicine & Health Sciences in Tempe, Arizona. She is the author of *Women's Encyclopedia of Natural Medicine.*

Across America, millions of women have been suffering for years from two common health problems that can be cured or at least dramatically improved.

If you're a woman with one of these conditions, you may mention it to your gynecologist, but chances are slim that you will get long-lasting relief from medication or other treatments prescribed by most MDs.

What I see in my practice: Every day, I treat women who are suffering unnecessarily from interstitial cystitis (also known as "painful bladder syndrome") and painful and/or lumpy breasts. Frequently, women actually give up on ever getting relief from these problems.

While anyone who has never endured these conditions may think that they are "not that big a deal," the truth is, these problems can greatly interfere with a woman's ability to go about her daily life and may even cause difficulties in her sexual relationship.

A natural approach: As a naturopathic physician, I look for the root cause of these conditions and help women use natural therapies that rely on the body's inherent ability to restore good health.

Here's how I treat my patients who have one of these vexing problems...

Interstitial Cystitis

Researchers are now finding that interstitial cystitis (IC) is much more prevalent than originally thought, affecting as many as eight million women in the US.

What it feels like: IC causes pelvic and/or perineal pain (the area between the anus and vagina). It can range from mild burning or discomfort to severe, debilitating pain that can also affect the bladder, lower abdomen, low back and/or thighs.

Along with the pain there can be urinary problems including a constant urge to urinate...frequent urination (more than eight times a day)...and needing to urinate several times overnight.

What MDs typically prescribe: Drugs, including painkillers, antidepressants and the medication pentosan (Elmiron), which is FDA approved for IC. Pentosan may take up to four months to relieve pain and six months to improve urinary frequency.

Other procedures, such as stretching the bladder and administering medication directly into the bladder, are sometimes also used.

All of these approaches have potential side effects, including gastrointestinal damage and liver problems and, most importantly, work less than 50% of the time.

My natural approach: Using several of the following natural treatments at the same time, my patients find that their symptoms of pain and urinary urgency and/or frequency typically improve within about three months—sometimes even faster.

Here's what I recommend...

•**Avoid acidic foods and beverages.** In one study, 53% of IC patients linked a flare-up of their symptoms to specific foods, especially citrus fruits, tomatoes, chocolate and acidic beverages such as alcohol and coffee. To see whether this is true for you, avoid these foods for two weeks. If your symptoms improve, avoid these foods indefinitely.

If you need more relief, try adding the following supplements (you may be able to reduce the doses as your symptoms start to improve)...*

•**Glycosaminoglycans (GAGs).** These two related natural compounds strengthen the lining of the bladder (epithelium), which may be more permeable in people with IC, leading to irritation and pain.

Typical dose: N-acetyl glucosamine—500 mg, twice daily...glucosamine sulfate—750 mg, twice daily.

•**Vitamin A.** This nutrient can help IC by decreasing inflammation and stimulating epithelial repair.

Typical dose: 5,000 international units (IU) daily.

•**L-arginine.** This amino acid helps regulate levels of nitric oxide in the blood, relaxing the muscles of the bladder and improving circulation. It also improves urinary frequency and sometimes helps reduce the pain associated with IC.

*Check with your doctor before starting a new supplement regimen—especially if you have a chronic medical condition and/or take medication.

Typical dose: 500 mg, twice daily.

•**Kava extract.** This herb from the South Pacific acts in several ways to relieve the symptoms of IC, including balancing potassium levels (high potassium can increase pain sensitivity).

Typical dose: One capsule, three times daily. Don't exceed 280 mg daily of kavalactones (an active ingredient).

Painful and/or Lumpy Breasts

Painful and/or lumpy breasts are one of the most common reasons women see a gynecologist. The good news is that this condition rarely accompanies breast cancer—cancer occurs as a painful, firm lump in only about 5% of cases.

What it feels like: Breasts that are painful and/or have one or more grape-size (or smaller) soft, rubbery lumps that can be moved are often due to hormonal changes during a woman's menstrual cycle. The breast pain can also be caused by an old injury or an acute infection (mastitis).

What MDs typically prescribe: When breasts are painful and/or lumpy due to hormonal changes, conventional doctors typically refer to it as fibrocystic breast disease.

Drug treatments that are frequently prescribed, such as birth control pills, can cause serious side effects, including headache, nausea and a slightly increased risk for stroke and deep vein thrombosis.

My natural approach: Because most women have some lumps or lumpy areas in their breasts all the time, as well as occasional pain, I don't consider this a disease.

Here's what I recommend…

•**Start with your diet.** Though scientists aren't sure why, research shows that simply eating more fruits and vegetables and avoiding caffeine (in all forms, including food sources such as chocolate and certain over-the-counter medications such as Anacin) can help prevent lumpy breasts.

In a one-year study, increasing daily soy intake also reduced breast tenderness and fibrocystic changes. Soy does not increase breast cancer risk, as some researchers had theorized, or pose danger to women who have had or have the disease.

Recommendation: One to two servings daily (a serving equals one cup of soy milk, for example, or four ounces of tofu). *Also, consider taking the following...*

•**Vitamin E.** Two studies show that vitamin E relieves breast pain and tenderness regardless of whether they are linked to a woman's menstrual cycle.

Typical dose: 400 IU to 800 IU daily of the d-alpha tocopherol form of vitamin E.

•**Evening primrose oil.** The linoleic and gamma linolenic acid in the oil help the body produce compounds that reduce pain and balance hormones.

Typical dose: 1,500 mg, twice daily.

If your condition doesn't improve in two to three months, consider…

•**Iodine.** Studies suggest that iodine deficiency plays a role in fibrocystic breasts. Without an adequate amount of iodine, breast tissue becomes more sensitive to estrogen, producing lumps.

Typical dose: 3 mg to 6 mg daily of aqueous iodine (by prescription).

Also helpful: Consume more iodine-rich foods, such as shellfish, seaweed, Swiss chard and lima beans.

Don't forget: In addition to undergoing an annual breast exam by a physician and any imaging tests he/she recommends, every woman should conduct a monthly breast self-exam. If any new, unusual changes, thickenings or lumps are detected, they should be promptly evaluated by a physician.

What to Eat for Underactive Thyroid

Pamela Wartian Smith, MD, MPH, MS, codirector of the Master's Program in Medical Sciences with a concentration in metabolic and nutritional medicine at Morsani College of Medicine, University of South Florida. Dr. Smith also is senior partner of the Michigan- and Florida-based Center for Personalized Medicine. She is author of *What You Must Know About Thyroid Disorders & What to Do About Them.* CenterForPersonalizedMedicine.com

D o you feel tired or cold much of the time? Are you anxious, irritable, depressed? Maybe you have trouble losing weight. If so, you may have an underactive thyroid (hypothyroidism)—and you're not alone. The American Association of Clinical Endocrinologists estimates that about 27 million adults (mostly women, but it also affects men), close to 10% of the population, suffer from thyroid disease. Hypothyroidism (underactive thyroid) is the most common form, accounting for about 90% of all cases.

What to do? Hormone replacement always is an option—but you might not need it.

My advice: Start with these lifestyle changes and other natural treatments. If you're currently taking thyroid medication, you may need less medication—so be sure to let your doctor know that you're taking these steps…

•**Add iodine.** You've probably heard that iodine deficiency is rare in the US because iodine is added to salt—and because many foods contain it. Not true. There's been an increase in iodine deficiency because many people avoid iodized salt (or are eating less salt in general). In addition, many people eat diets that are high in pasta and bread. These foods often contain bromide, a compound that decreases iodine absorption.

My advice: Get tested for iodine. Low levels are easily corrected by using iodized salt...eating sea vegetables (such as nori) a few times a week...or by taking an iodine supplement.

Important: Don't take an iodine supplement unless you need it. Too much iodine can cause thyroid inflammation and increase your risk of developing Hashimoto's thyroiditis (a kind of hypothyroidism) or thyroid cancer.

•**Eat Brazil nuts.** They're high in selenium, a mineral that helps the body convert thyroxine (T4, a less active form of thyroid hormone) to triiodothyronine (T3, the active form). One study found that low-thyroid patients given selenium supplements later tested normal on a thyroid test. A few Brazil nuts a day will provide enough selenium. Other high-selenium foods include fish, chicken, turkey and beef.

Note: If you live in North Dakota or South Dakota, then you already have a lot of selenium in your diet because the ground in these states is rich in selenium. Therefore, you probably will not need additional selenium as a food or supplement.

•**Take probiotics.** I recommend them for everyone with low-thyroid function. Studies have shown that probiotic supplements—Lactobacillus, Bifidobacterium, etc.—improve the body's ability to absorb the nutrients that are needed for thyroid health. I've had patients who were able to avoid using medication simply by optimizing their digestive health with probiotics.

My advice: Buy probiotic supplements that contain at least 20 billion colony-forming units per dose (available at health-food stores and pharmacies). Research has shown that people tend to do better when they rotate bacterial strains about every six months.

•**Take a daily multi.** Many different nutrients are required for the body to convert T4 to the more active form of thyroid hormone, T3. Even if you eat a nutritious diet, you might not be getting enough. For insurance, take a multinutrient supplement that includes all the basics, such as potassium, selenium, B vitamins and zinc. Ask your health-care provider if you need iron in your multivitamin.

●**Don't skip breakfast.** The pancreas ramps up insulin production in the morning and again in the evening. You need to synchronize meals with high-insulin times to improve insulin sensitivity—the ability of cells to respond to insulin and absorb blood sugar. One study found that people with improved insulin sensitivity had lower TSH (see box on the right) and higher T4. An example of a good breakfast would be turkey sausage and berries. The sausage is a protein that slows the absorption of the carbohydrate (the berries), which is better for blood sugar levels.

●**Avoid harmful foods and ingredients.** Sugar, refined carbohydrates (such as white bread and white rice) and soft drinks can contribute to hypothyroidism by decreasing the levels of important minerals in your body. Opt for healthier choices—a Mediterranean-style diet is ideal, along with plenty of purified water.

If Your Symptoms Don't Improve...

If your symptoms don't improve from lifestyle changes and natural treatments, you'll probably need a thyroid medication. The good

---

Don't Trust the Thyroid Test

The standard test for low thyroid might not provide a clear answer. You could test normal but still have thyroid function that's at the lower end of the range—which, for some people, is enough to cause problems.

Low thyroid is diagnosed with a simple blood test for thyroid-stimulating hormone (TSH). If you have low thyroxine, a thyroid hormone, your body will produce high levels of TSH to compensate. People with significantly elevated TSH—say, a reading of 5.0 mIU/L (milli-international units per liter) or higher—have obvious hypothyroidism.

What if you test within a normal range but still are having symptoms? It doesn't mean you're imagining things. Laboratories have different reference ranges, the measurements that are considered normal. In 2004, endocrinologists suggested a change in the normal range so that a TSH reading of 2.5 was the upper limit. But for some people, normal isn't optimal. I've found that patients can suffer from thyroid-related symptoms even when they "pass" the TSH test.

This is why it is very important to have a complete thyroid panel done when you see your doctor and not just a TSH and free T4. An entire thyroid panel includes TSH, free T3, free T4, reverse T3 and thyroid antibodies.

---

thing about these prescription drugs is that they precisely mimic the effects of your body's natural hormones. You're unlikely to experience any side effects after your doctor has determined the correct dose. Until then, you might have the same symptoms that you had before (if you're taking too little). Or, you might have shakiness, insomnia, rapid heartbeat or an increased appetite (if you're taking too much).

The standard prescription hormones, such as Synthroid or Levothroid, contain only T4.

My advice: Ask your doctor to prescribe one of the powdered thyroid hormones—such as Armour Thyroid, Euthroid or Liotrix—that contains T3 along with T4. They usually come in a standard ratio of four parts T4 to one part T3. Studies have shown that most patients who are given both tend to do better than those who take only T4.

Yin/Yang Way to Eat to Stop Hot Flashes

Laurie Steelsmith, ND, is the author of *Natural Choices for Women's Health* and a medical reviewer for *HealthyWoman from Bottom Line.* Her private practice in naturopathic and Chinese medicine is in Honolulu. NaturalChoicesForWomen.com

When in the throes of a menopausal hot flash, we should rightly be given permission to strip naked and jump into a snowbank. For relief, conventional doctors often recommend hormone therapy, but it has been linked to an increased risk for breast cancer, heart disease and stroke—and a recent study found that users had a 29% greater risk for ovarian cancer than nonusers.

You can minimize hot flashes by avoiding foods that are "warming"—a classification that, surprisingly, has nothing to do with the temperature at which a food is served and often is not based on its level of spiciness. Rather, warming foods are those with a lot of yang or "hot energy."

According to traditional Chinese medicine, yin and yang are opposites or counterparts that exist everywhere in the universe. Yin is associated with cold, quiet, passivity, water and nighttime...yang is associated with heat, noise, activity, fire and daytime. Women tend to have more yin, while men tend to have more yang. At menopause, yin gets depleted—in fact, estrogen and progesterone are both cooling yin hormones—leaving an excess of yang. Stress exacerbates hot flashes because stress hormones such as cortisol are yang. Warming foods, which have more yang than yin, promote hot flashes because they create more of a yin/yang disparity than you already have.

A food is deemed yin or yang based on centuries of tradition, the food's innate traits and how it makes the body feel—not necessarily on whether it is hot or cold. The classification system is sometimes somewhat intuitive. For example, meat generally is more yang than fruits and vegetables (since mammals are warm-blooded and mobile while plants are cool and stationary). Some plant foods are more yin than others—for instance, lettuce (which is soft and spoils quickly) is more yin than a carrot (which is hard and lasts a long time). Warming foods tend to grow in colder climates and vice versa, so a peach is more yang than a papaya.

But: Sometimes there is no clear rationale. For instance, although trout is said to be particularly yang, many other types of seafood are not...and while most spices are yang, salt and a few others are yin.

Admittedly, this gets complicated—so instead of trying to figure out or remember which foods are yang, just print this article and post it in your pantry. You don't want to avoid all yang foods since many are nutritious, but with trial and error you'll see which ones trigger your hot flashes and which are OK for you.

Yang Foods to Limit...

Fruits: Cherries...coconuts...guavas...kumquats...lemons...lychees...peaches...raspberries.

Vegetables: Cauliflower...mustard greens...onions...pumpkins...scallions.

Grains/nuts/seeds: Chestnuts...pine nuts...pumpkin seeds...sticky (glutinous) rice...walnuts.

Dairy: Butter...goat's milk...yogurt.

Meat/poultry/seafood: Anchovies...chicken...crayfish...lamb...lobster...mussels...shrimp...trout...venison.

Herbs/spices: Anise...basil...caraway...cardamom...chives...cinnamon...cloves...coriander...dill...fennel...garlic...ginger...nutmeg...pepper...rosemary...saffron...thyme...turmeric.

Miscellaneous: Alcohol...brown sugar...coffee...molasses...soybean oil...vinegar.

Regular consumption of cooling foods that are more yin can reduce the number and severity of hot flashes (though eating them during a hot flash won't have a quick enough effect to halt your heat wave). When you do eat a yang food, counterbalance its effects by having a cooling yin food at the same time.

Yin Foods to Keep You Cool...

Fruits: Bananas...grapefruit...kiwifruit...loquats...melon...mulberries...oranges...papayas...pears...persimmons...plums...pomegranates...strawberries...tangerines.

Vegetables: Alfalfa sprouts...asparagus...bamboo shoots...broccoli...burdock root...cabbage...celery...cucumbers...eggplant...lettuce...lotus root...kelp...mung beans...mushrooms...nori...radishes...spinach...summer squash...sweet potatoes...tomatoes...turnips...watercress.

Grains/nuts/seeds: Barley...buckwheat...millet...wheat...wheat bran.

Seafood: Clams...crab...octopus.

Herbs/spices: Green tea...marjoram...peppermint...salt.

Miscellaneous: Sesame oil...soy sauce...tofu...water.

Neutral Foods

Many other foods are fairly equally balanced in yin and yang. These are unlikely to affect hot flashes one way or the other. *Neutral foods include...*

Fruits: Apricots...figs...grapes...pineapple...red dates.

Vegetables: Beets...carrots...olives...peas...potatoes...string beans...yams.

Grains/nuts/seeds: Almonds...corn...hazelnuts...oats...peanuts...rice...rye...sesame seeds...sunflower seeds.

Dairy: Cheese...cow's milk.

Meat/poultry/seafood: Beef...duck...ham...oysters...pork...sardines...white fish.

Miscellaneous: Eggs...honey...white sugar.

Cool Hot Flashes with Rhubarb Extract

Mark A. Stengler, NMD, a naturopathic doctor and founder of the Stengler Center for Integrative Medicine in Encinitas, California. He is author or coauthor of numerous books, including *The Natural Physician's Healing Therapies* and *Bottom Line's Prescription for Natural Cures,* and author of the newsletter *Health Revelations.* MarkStengler.com

The health benefits of rhubarb have long been recognized. Now German researchers are investigating the use of an extract derived from rhubarb to cool the hot flashes of perimenopause and menopause.

In their newest study, they found that ERr 731, the name of the extract derived from rhubarb, significantly reduced the number and intensity of hot flashes in perimenopausal women, compared with women who were taking a placebo. The women took one tablet of ERr 731 daily for 12 weeks.

Scientists don't fully understand how or why this rhubarb extract works, but it does contain a unique phytoestrogen (naturally occurring chemical in plants that acts like estrogen), which is a possible key to its efficacy. No harmful side effects have been associated with the extract.

Brand to try: Estrovera, a tablet that has ERr 731. Distributed by Metagenics (800-692-9400, Metagenics.com), it is available through health-care professionals and online. (A list of practitioners by region is available on the manufacturer's website.)

Medicinal Asparagus for Fertility

Mark A. Stengler, NMD, a naturopathic doctor and founder of the Stengler Center for Integrative Medicine in Encinitas, California. He is author or coauthor of numerous books, including *The Natural Physician's Healing Therapies* and *Bottom Line's Prescription for Natural Cures*, and author of the newsletter *Health Revelations*. MarkStengler.com

Asparagus is a nutritional powerhouse that has long been known for its medicinal properties. Asparagus is available year-round, but it is in season in spring and summer.

Medicinal properties: In traditional Indian medicine, asparagus is used to strengthen the female reproductive system. The Chinese believe that asparagus roots (dried or raw as an herbal medication) spur feelings of compassion and love.

The science behind these beliefs: Asparagus root contains compounds called steroidal glycosides that can affect hormone production and possibly influence emotions.

Nutritional benefits: Asparagus delivers potassium, folate, vitamin K, the compound rutin (which helps to protect blood vessels) and the anti-inflammatory flavonoid quercetin. One cup of cooked asparagus (about eight medium-sized spears) provides 3.6 grams of fiber—all with only 40 calories.

To enjoy: The tastiest part of an asparagus spear (whether thin or thick) is near the tip. The part farthest away from the tip is woody, fibrous and not tasty, which is why it's commonly cut off. Asparagus can be eaten raw or cooked. (There is not much nutritional difference.)

Some people have naturally occurring enzymes in their digestive tracts that break down sulfur-containing amino acids in asparagus resulting in smelly urine, which is temporary and goes away on its own.

If you have gout, don't eat asparagus—a chemical in it, purine, may aggravate that condition.

Ways to use: In addition to preparing it as a side dish (with garlic or ginger), add steamed or stir-fried asparagus to scrambled eggs or to pasta with garlic and olive oil.

Herbs and Supplements That Relieve Lupus Symptoms

Sara Korsunsky, ND, is a licensed doctor of naturopathic medicine with a family-oriented private practice at the Centre for Natural Medicine in Winnipeg, Manitoba, Canada. Since her diagnosis with lupus at the age of 16, Dr. Korsunsky has used naturopathic and conventional medicine to maintain a full and balanced life with a chronic illness. NaturalMedicine.mb.ca

An autoimmune disorder, lupus affects women eight times more often than men. There is no known cure, so treatment focuses on minimizing the disease's symptoms, such as skin rashes, fatigue, fever, gastrointestinal upset, and muscle and joint pain. I've been able to reduce my list of lupus symptoms from 10 to just three and now I experience only occasional, very mild flares. I've maintained my health this way for several years now—even through a pregnancy, a time when lupus symptoms typically worsen. Many of my patients with lupus also have seen huge improvements by following these treatment guidelines.

Prescription lupus drugs (such as corticosteroids, nonsteroidal anti-inflammatories and immunosuppressants) may offer quicker symptom relief, but natural approaches generally have fewer side effects and bring about better overall health in the long run. For maximum effectiveness and safety, it is vital to work directly with a qualified naturopathic doctor who can customize your treatment. Autoimmune diseases manifest differently in different patients, and there are significant individual variations in body chemistry, diet and lifestyle.

Important: Do not stop taking your lupus medication on your own…and do not start taking supplements before checking with your doctor, as some supplements may cause side effects or stimulate your already overactive immune system. *Instead, talk with your doctor about complementing your conventional care with natural supplements that help to…*

•**Quell inflammation.** Because lupus is a systemic inflammatory disease, it can affect just about any part of the body—skin, joints, muscles, organs. My number-one recommendation is to supplement with omega-3 fatty acids (as fish oil) to help keep inflammation under control. Also potentially beneficial are flaxseed oil…antioxidants such as vitamins C and E…and the anti-inflammatory spices turmeric and ginger, which are available in capsule form.

•**Support digestion.** Nausea, constipation and other gastrointestinal problems are common among lupus patients because digestive function is strongly linked to immune function…and because nonsteroidal anti-inflammatory drugs can damage the gut wall. Supplementing with digestive enzymes, such as bromelain (which comes from the stem of the pineapple plant), can improve digestion.

•**Increase energy and improve adrenal function.** Lupus patients often feel fatigued due to underfunctioning of the adrenal glands. Also, the steroid drug prednisone, which many patients take, can worsen fatigue by further suppressing adrenal function. Helpful: A multivitamin (particularly important are vitamins A, D and E)…an additional vitamin B complex supplement (since a multivitamin may not provide optimal amounts of the B vitamins needed for lupus)…and the herbs licorice root and ashwagandha.

Herbal Relief for Painful Mouth Sores

Eric Yarnell, ND, is an associate professor in the department of botanical medicine at Bastyr University in Kenmore, Washington, and a private practitioner at Northwest Naturopathic Urology in Seattle. He is the author or coauthor of 10 books on natural medicine, including *Nature's Cures: What You Should Know.*

The inside of your mouth hurts like crazy, so you stand in front of a mirror and open wide. Do you see white, lacy, raised patches…red, swollen, tender spots…and/or open sores? If so, you may have oral lichen planus (LIE-kun PLAY-nus), an inflammatory disease that affects more women than men and often arises in middle age. Lesions usually appear on the inside of the cheeks but also may develop on the tongue, gums, inner lips and throat. The disorder causes burning pain…a metallic taste in the mouth…sensitivity to spicy foods…dry mouth…and/or bleeding gums.

Oral lichen planus is not contagious. It occurs when the immune system attacks the cells of the mucous membranes in the mouth. The exact reason for this attack is unknown, but outbreaks can be triggered by allergies (for instance, to a food or dental product)…a viral infection (such as hepatitis C)…certain vaccines and medications (including nonsteroidal anti-inflammatory drugs)…or stress.

When outbreaks are linked to an allergy or drug, identifying and avoiding the offending substance can resolve the problem. However, in many cases, oral lichen planus is a chronic condition in which flare-ups continue to come and go indefinitely, with lesions lasting for days, weeks or even months. Since there is no known cure, treatment focuses on alleviating discomfort.

Problem: Steroid medication helps, but has potentially serious side effects. Topical steroids can lead to thrush (a fungal infection of the mouth) and suppress adrenal gland function, while oral and injected steroids increase the risk for osteoporosis, diabetes, high blood pressure and high cholesterol. And once steroid treatment is halted, lesions may return.

Intriguing alternative: Herbs. While the herbs below have not been proven to cure oral lichen planus, they can ease discomfort... and some patients who use herbal treatments experience quick resolution of symptoms and remain free of recurrences for long periods of time.

Important: Certain herbs can have side effects, so work with a health-care provider knowledgeable about herbal medicines, such as a naturopathic doctor, who can devise a safe and effective protocol for you and determine appropriate dosages. A swish-and-swallow approach (taking a mouthful of a diluted herbal extract and swishing it in the mouth before swallowing it) is usually most effective. The herb acts topically as well as systemically—your own practitioner can advise you on this. You can use one or more of the following herbs, depending on the specific symptom (or symptoms) that bothers you most. *Ask your health-care provider about using the following...*

•**For pain—aloe vera (***Aloe barbadensis***).** The gel found inside the leaves of the aloe plant contain complex carbohydrates, including glucomannan, that soothe painful tissues and modulate the immune response.

•**For inflammation—turmeric (***Curcuma longa***).** This spice contains substances called curcuminoids that reduce inflammation via multiple pathways. It doesn't dissolve well in water, so try dissolving turmeric in milk.

Caution: People who are prone to kidney stones should not use turmeric (which is high in oxalic acid)—for them, curcumin extract is better.

•**For easily irritated tissues—tormentil (***Potentilla tormentilla***).** Used in the form of a tincture (a medicinal extract in a solution of alcohol), this herbal preparation coats lesions, protecting them from irritation by food or compounds in saliva. This remedy should not be used within 30 minutes of taking any other medications, as the herb may block absorption of other drugs.

Caution: People who want to avoid alcohol should not use tormentil.

•**For stress—licorice root (***Glycyrrhiza glabra***) or deglycyrrhizinated licorice (DGL).** This is an adaptogen that helps patients handle the anxiety and stress that can contribute to oral lichen planus...it also modulates the immune system. It often is used in tincture form, though patients who want to avoid alcohol should use chewable DGL tablets instead.

Caution: Licorice root remedies should not be used by patients who have uncontrolled hypertension or who are taking corticosteroids or other drugs that can deplete potassium.

Note: Oral lichen planus may increase the risk for oral cancers, get regular oral cancer screenings from a doctor or dentist.

CHAPTER 12

Superfoods for Men's Health

Food That Fixes ED

John La Puma, MD, board-certified specialist in internal medicine and trained chef with a private nutritional medical practice in Santa Barbara, California, and cofounder of the popular video series ChefMD. He is author of *Refuel: A 24-Day Eating Plan to Shed Fat, Boost Testosterone, and Pump Up Strength and Stamina.* DrJohnLaPuma.com

Study titled "Dietary flavonoid intake and incidence of erectile dysfunction" by researchers at Norwich Medical School, University of East Anglia, United Kingdom, Harvard T.H. Chan School of Public Health, Boston, Brigham and Women's Hospital, Boston, Harvard Medical School, Boston, published in *The American Journal of Clinical Nutrition.*

M en: If you like to eat blueberries, you may beat the odds of developing erectile dysfunction (ED). It also helps if you eat strawberries, oranges, grapefruit, apples and pears—and drink red wine.

So suggests a recent study. But ED can be caused by some serious health issues. Could a handful of berries really be that powerful?

The Flavonoid Boost

In the study, Harvard researchers analyzed the diets and ED symptoms of 25,000 men in the Health Professionals Follow-Up Study. In the period that this analysis focused on, the men were in their 50s, 60s and 70s and older. The researchers focused on phytochemicals called flavonoids—and the foods, mostly fruits, that are the biggest source of them in the American diet.

Results: Men whose diets were higher in these flavonoid-rich fruits were 14% less likely to develop ED over a 10-year period. Citrus fruits were a major flavonoid contributor. (Dark chocolate and soy foods, both of which are also flavonoid-rich, were not studied in this analysis.)

Blueberries stood out. In a separate analysis, men who ate them more than three times a week, on average, were 22% less likely to develop ED.

What's so special about flavonoids? Berries here are acting in the same way as Viagra, but they're a lot cheaper and they taste better. In animal studies, flavonoids inhibit a biological pathway that makes the penis flaccid...and boost production of nitric oxide, which facilitates erections during sexual activity. In one study of rats with diabetes and ED, for example, adding a specific flavonoid (quercetin) to their chow actually reversed ED.

Medications such as *sildenafil* (Viagra) work through similar mechanisms, but unlike blueberries, they don't promote heart health—and they have side effects.

To be sure, no one is saying that you can pop a few blueberries in your mouth, wait a half-hour and jump into the sack. The study unveiled not a quick fix but a long-term benefit of a flavonoid-rich diet. The good news: While you're saving your sexual function, you're likely saving your heart, too.

Beyond Prevention

The diet connection makes sense when you realize that erectile dysfunction often is a cardiovascular problem. The penile artery is about half the width of the coronary artery, so inflammation there creates symptoms first. Men with ED have cardiac disease until proven otherwise—it's an early warning sign.

That's why a heart-healthy diet is so important for prevention—and even treatment—of ED. In one study, he notes, men with ED who ate three ounces of heart-healthy flavonoid-rich pistachios for three weeks had improvement in their symptoms. Another study found that flavonoid-rich walnuts, like blueberries, boost nitric oxide production. A number of studies have shown that the dietary pattern, especially a Mediterranean diet...along with other interventions such as quitting smoking and increased physical activity...can be both preventive and therapeutic.

Another Notch in the Blueberry Belt

On the other hand, if you're looking for just one food to add to your diet to improve your health, and perhaps help preserve your sexual vitality, you can't go wrong with blueberries.

It's not just men who benefit. Blueberries are good for brain health in both men and women, improving cognitive function and memory in older adults.

And if any women are reading this article, there's a heart benefit for you, too. The same Harvard group that discovered the ED connection reported a few years ago that women who consumed at least three servings of blueberries or strawberries a week were 34% less likely to get heart disease.

Blueberries—quite a sexy food indeed.

Foods That Relieve Prostate Pain

Mark A. Stengler, NMD, a naturopathic doctor and founder of the Stengler Center for Integrative Medicine in Encinitas, California. He is author or coauthor of numerous books, including *The Natural Physician's Healing Therapies* and *Bottom Line's Prescription for Natural Cures*, and author of the newsletter *Health Revelations*. MarkStengler.com

When it comes to men's health, we hear a lot about enlarged prostate and prostate cancer. But there is another prostate ailment that gets much less attention yet affects many men. Prostatitis, a very painful condition, is inflammation of the prostate gland. It can be difficult to diagnose because its symptoms (persistent pain in the pelvis or rectum...discomfort in the abdomen, lower back, penis or testicles...difficult, painful or frequent urination or painful ejaculation) are similar to those of other conditions such as an enlarged prostate or a urinary tract infection.

It is estimated that almost half of all men will be affected by prostatitis at some point in their lives. If the condition lasts for three months or longer, it's considered to be chronic prostatitis.

Mainstream medicine often is unsuccessful in treating chronic prostatitis, leaving men in pain and without hope of feeling better. In my practice, I have had lots of success treating chronic prostatitis as both an inflammatory condition (which it always is) and as a possible fungal infection.

Reasons Behind Prostatitis

For a long time, it was thought that prostatitis could be caused only by bacterial infection. That view was dispelled when several studies found that the bacteria in the prostates of both healthy men and men with prostatitis were essentially identical. It's now understood that most prostatitis cases are not caused by bacteria. Still, most mainstream physicians routinely prescribe antibiotics for it—a treatment that is appropriate only if your case is one of a very small number actually caused by bacteria.

Although prostate inflammation is not well understood, the inflammation could be the result of inadequate fluid drainage into the prostatic ducts...an abnormal immune response...or a fungal infection.

Prostatitis Treatment Plan

If you experience any of the symptoms of prostatitis mentioned above, see your doctor. Your visit should include a rectal exam to check for swelling or tenderness in the prostate...and a laboratory test of prostatic fluid to check for bacterial infection. (Fluid is released during prostate gland massage.) I also recommend that you have your doctor order a urine culture to test for fungal infection (most medical doctors don't test for this).

In a small number of cases, the lab test does reveal a bacterial infection, and an antibiotic is appropriately prescribed. But if there is no bacterial infection, then I recommend that men with this condition follow an anti-inflammatory, antifungal treatment plan for two months. If symptoms subside but don't disappear, continue for another two months. Even if you don't have a test for fungal infection, I often advise following the antifungal portion of the program (along with the inflammation portion) to see if it helps to relieve symptoms.

Foods That Battle Prostatitis

Anti-inflammatory diet. If you are thinking, Why is Dr. Stengler telling me again about an anti-inflammatory diet?—I'm telling you because it works. Eating a diet of whole foods and cutting out packaged and processed foods go a long way to reducing inflammation in general and prostate inflammation in particular.

Eat: A variety of plant products to maximize your intake of antioxidants, which are natural anti-inflammatories...coldwater fish such as salmon, trout and sardines, which are high in omega-3 fatty acids...and pumpkin seeds, which are high in zinc, a mineral that helps reduce prostate swelling.

Don't eat: Foods that are high in saturated fat, such as red meat and dairy, which can make inflammation worse. Avoid alcohol, caffeine, refined sugar and trans fats, all of which tend to contribute to inflammation.

•**Antifungal diet.** If you already are following the anti-inflammatory diet above, then you have eliminated refined sugar from your diet. (Fungi thrive on sugar!) Also try eliminating all grains (including whole grains and rice) from your diet. Fungi thrive on these foods.

Prostate-Protective Supplements

The following supplements have targeted benefits for prostate inflammation. They are safe to take together, and there are no side effects. Many men feel much better within two weeks of taking these supplements.

•**Rye pollen extract.** Studies show that rye pollen extract can relieve the pain of chronic prostatitis. In one study published in *British Journal of Urology*, men with chronic prostatitis took three tablets of rye pollen extract daily. After six months, 36% had no more symptoms and 42% reported symptom improvement. Follow label instructions. The pollen component in rye pollen does not contain gluten, but if you have celiac disease or a severe allergy to gluten, look for a certified gluten-free product.

•**Quercetin.** This powerful flavonoid helps reduce prostate inflammation. *Dose:* 1,000 milligrams (mg) twice daily.

•**Fish oil.** In addition to eating anti-inflammatory foods, these supplements are a rich source of inflammation-fighting omega-3 fatty acids. *Dose:* 2,000 mg daily of combined EPA and DHA.

Antifungal Supplements

Many patients benefit from taking one or more antifungal remedies. Several herbs—such as oregano, pau d'arco, garlic and grapefruit seed extract—have potent antifungal properties. They are available in capsule and liquid form. For doses, follow label instructions. Most patients feel better within two to four weeks of taking antifungal supplements.

What You Eat Affects Your Prostate

Geo Espinosa, ND, a naturopathic doctor and expert in prostate cancer and men's health. He is founder and director of the Integrative and Functional Urology Center at New York University's Langone Medical Center in New York City. Dr. Espinosa is the author of *THRIVE Don't Only Survive! Dr. Geo's Guide to Living Your Best Life Before & After Prostate Cancer* and coauthor of *Bottom Line's 1,000 Cures for 200 Ailments.* DrGeo.com

Two studies published in 2016 showed how crucial food choices are for prostate health.

Study I: Drinking sugary beverages (including not only sodas and sweetened iced tea but also fruit juices) was linked to a three times greater risk for prostate cancer...and eating processed lunch foods (such as pizza and hamburgers) doubled prostate cancer risk.

Study II: Among men who had already been diagnosed with prostate cancer, those who ate lots of saturated fats (found in fatty red meats, cheese and butter) were more likely to have the most aggressive form of the disease...but men who ate diets that emphasized fish and nuts—high in polyunsaturated fats—had less aggressive prostate cancer.

Bottom line on diet: Eat a diet that is rich in fruits, vegetables, nuts, fish, legumes and whole grains...and limit saturated fats, processed foods and sugary beverages.

CHAPTER 13

Anti-Aging Foods

Six Herbs That Slow Aging

Donald R. Yance, CN, MH, RH (AHG), clinical master herbalist and certified nutrition-ist. He is medical director at the Mederi Foundation's Centre for Natural Healing in Ashland, Oregon…founder and president of the Mederi Foundation, a not-for-profit organization for professional education and clinical research in collaborative medi-cine…and president and formulator of Natura Health Products. He is author of *Adaptogens in Medical Herbalism* and *Herbal Medicine, Healing & Cancer.* DonnieYance.com

You can't escape aging. But many Americans are aging prematurely. *Surprising fact:* The US ranks 42nd out of 191 countries in life expectancy, according to the Census Bureau and the National Center for Health Statistics.

The leading cause of this rapid, premature aging is chronic stress. Stress is any factor, positive or negative, that requires the body to make a response or change to adapt. It can be psychological stress, including the modern addiction to nonstop stimulation and speed. Or it can be physiological stress—such as eating a highly processed diet…sitting for hours every day…absorbing toxins from food, water and air…and spending time in artificial light.

Chronic stress overwhelms the body's homeostasis, its inborn ability to adapt to stress and stay balanced, strong and healthy. The result?

Your hormonal and immune systems are weakened. Inflammation flares up, damaging cells. Daily energy decreases, fatigue increases, and you can't manage life as effectively. You suffer from one or more illnesses, take several medications and find yourself in a downward spiral of worsening health. Even though you might live to be 75 or older, you're surviving, not thriving.

We can reduce stress by making lifestyle changes such as eating better and exercising. You also can help beat stress and slow aging with adaptogens. These powerful herbs balance and strengthen the hormonal and immune systems... give you more energy...and repair cellular damage—thereby boosting your body's ability to adapt to chronic stress.

Important: Adaptogens are generally safe, but always talk with your doctor before taking any supplement.

Here are six of the most powerful adaptogens...

●**Ashwagandha.**

This adaptogen from Ayurveda (the ancient system of natural healing from India) can help with a wide range of conditions.

Main actions: It is energizing and improves sleep, and it can help with arthritis, anxiety, depression, dementia and respiratory disorders, such as asthma, bronchitis and emphysema.

Important benefit: It is uniquely useful for cancer—it can help kill cancer cells...reduce the toxicity of chemotherapy (and prevent resistance to chemotherapeutic drugs)...relieve cancer-caused fatigue...and prevent recurrence.

●**Eleuthero.**

This is the most well-researched adaptogen (with more than 3,000 published studies). It often is called the "king" of adaptogens. (It was introduced in the US as "Siberian ginseng," but it is not a ginseng.)

Main actions: Along with providing energy and vitality, eleuthero protects the body against the ill effects of any kind of stress, such as extremes of heat or cold, excessive exercise and radiation. More than any other adaptogen, it helps normalize any type of physiological abnormality—including high or low blood pressure...and high or low blood sugar.

Important benefit: Eleuthero is a superb "ergogenic" (performance-enhancing) aid that can help anyone involved in sports improve strength and endurance and recover from injury.

●**Ginseng.**

Used as a traditional medicine in Asia for more than 5,000 years and the subject of more than 500 scientific papers, ginseng has two primary species—*Panax ginseng* (Korean or Asian ginseng) and *Panax quinquefolius* (American ginseng).

Main actions: Ginseng is antifatigue and antiaging. It increases muscle strength and endurance and improves reaction times. It also strengthens the immune system and the heart and helps regulate blood sugar.

Important benefits: American ginseng can be beneficial for recovering from the common cold, pneumonia or bronchitis (particularly with a dry cough)...and chronic stress accompanied by depression or anxiety.

Korean or Asian ginseng is helpful for increasing physical performance, especially endurance and energy. It is effective for restoring adrenal function and neurological health such as learning and memory.

•Rhaponticum.

This herb contains more anabolic (strengthening and muscle-building) compounds than any other plant. It is my number-one favorite herb for increasing stamina and strength.

Main actions: It normalizes the central nervous and cardiovascular systems...improves sleep, appetite and mood...and increases the ability to work and function under stressful conditions.

Important benefit: This herb is wonderful for anyone recovering from injury, trauma or surgery.

•Rhodiola.

Rhodiola has gained popularity over the past few years as studies show that it rivals eleuthero and ginseng as an adaptogen. It is widely used by Russian athletes to increase energy.

Main actions: Rhodiola increases blood supply to the muscles and the brain, enhancing physical and mental performance, including memory. It normalizes the cardiovascular system and protects the heart from stress. It also strengthens immunity.

Red flag: Don't use rhodiola alone—it is extremely astringent and drying. It is best used along with other adaptogens in a formula.

•Schisandra.

This herb has a long history of use as an adaptogen in China, Russia, Japan, Korea and Tibet. The fruit is commonly used, but the seed is more powerful.

Main actions: Schisandra can treat stress-induced fatigue...protect and detoxify the liver...treat insomnia, depression and vision problems...and enhance athletic performance.

Important benefit: This adaptogen may help night vision—one study showed it improved adaptation to darkness by 90%.

Combinations Are Best

Any one herb has limitations in its healing power. But a combination or formula of adaptogenic herbs overcomes those limitations—because the adaptogens act in concert, making them more powerful.

This concept of synergy—multiple herbs acting together are more effective than one herb acting alone—is key to the effectiveness of the herbal formulas of traditional Chinese medicine (TCM) and Ayurveda. Both these ancient forms of medicine often employ a dozen or more herbs in their formulas.

But it's not only the combination of herbs that makes them effective—it's also the quality of the herbs. There are many more poor-quality adaptogens on the market than high-quality (or even mediocre-quality).

My advice: Look for an herbalist or herbal company that knows all about the source and content of the herbs it uses. Example: Herbalist & Alchemist, a company that grows most of the herbs used in its products.

Or find a product sold to health practitioners, who then sell it to their patients—this type of product is more likely to be high quality. *Example:* MediHerb, from Standard Process.

Herbal formulas from my company, Natura Health Products, also meet these criteria for high quality.

Why You Should Eat Soy...

Mark Messina, PhD, associate professor of nutrition at Loma Linda University in Loma Linda, California, and former program director with the diet and cancer branch of National Cancer Institute. He is an internationally recognized expert on soy and co-author of *The Simple Soybean and Your Health.*

Soy is one of the few foods permitted by the US Food and Drug Administration (FDA) to include a health claim on the label. The claim states that diets low in saturated fat and cholesterol that include 25 grams of soy protein a day may reduce the risk of heart disease.

Evidence suggests that soy may be helpful for a range of other diseases, including osteoporosis and some kinds of cancer. However, other studies suggest that it may increase the risk of breast cancer. *Here's what you need to know...*

Soy Benefits for You

Preliminary research suggests that soy may be helpful for the following conditions…

●**Cardiovascular disease.** The Japanese consume an average of 11 grams of soy protein per day per person—and the rate of heart disease in Japan is among the lowest in the world. (Americans average two grams of soy per day.) *How soy helps…*

●Soy protein lowers LDL (bad) cholesterol by 4% to 5%—more when it is a substitute for red meat or other dietary sources of saturated fat. Soy protein may increase the activity of cellular receptors that "trap" LDL and take it out of circulation.

●Soy is rich in isoflavones, a class of chemical compounds that act like weaker versions of the hormone estrogen. Isoflavones, known as phytoestrogens, enhance the ability of arteries to relax and/or dilate, improving blood flow. This is true for men and women.

●Soy lowers blood pressure by as much as 15 points, according to some studies. Other studies, however, have shown more modest or no effects.

●Soy has linolenic acid, which may reduce heart disease mortality by 20%.

●**Prostate cancer.** Japanese men have significantly less incidence of prostate cancer than American men, possibly due to soy. A study of cancer patients found that levels of prostate-specific antigen (PSA), an indicator of prostate cancer, leveled off in men given soy isoflavones for six months. Isoflavones are believed to inhibit enzymes that fuel tumor growth.

Most men will develop prostate cancer at some point in their lives. This cancer grows slowly, so most men never have related health problems—but prostate cancer still is the second-leading cause of cancer deaths among men (lung cancer is the first). I advise every man to eat soy.

●**Menopausal discomfort.** The phyto-estrogens in soy are metabolized in the body into equol, an estrogenlike compound. Soy seems to be most effective for women who experience five or more hot flashes a day—it can reduce hot-flash frequency by up to 40%. Some menopausal women who eat soy also notice an improvement in vaginal dryness.

●**Diabetic renal disease.** One of the most serious complications of diabetes is kidney disease, which can lead to kidney failure. Substituting soy for animal protein lowers the glomerular filtration rate, a measure of kidney stress, and may slow kidney damage.

Studies Needed

Soy may be helpful for the following conditions, but research so far is inconclusive...

•**Osteoporosis.** Soy has been promoted for bone strength on the mistaken premise that Asian women have less incidence of osteoporosis than American women. Not true. While their rate of hip fractures is lower than in the US, the Japanese have twice the rate of vertebral fractures. The difference in hip fractures probably is due to a difference in anatomy, which makes the hip less likely to break on impact.

Other evidence suggests that isoflavones do promote bone strength. The USDA and the National Institutes of Health (NIH) currently are allotting significant resources—about $10 million—for studies to determine whether isoflavones play a role in bone health.

•**Breast cancer.** Asian studies indicate that women who eat soy foods three or more times weekly have a reduced risk of breast cancer.

However, some researchers believe that soy may increase the risk of breast cancer. Most breast tumors are stimulated by estrogen. A diet high in isoflavones, which mimic some of estrogen's effects, could stimulate tumor growth in women with these estrogen-positive tumors.

Animal studies at the University of Illinois found that isoflavones increased tumor growth—yet similar studies at Harvard showed the opposite. No one knows if soy isoflavones have any effect on breast cancer in humans. A recent two-year study of premenopausal women found that soy had no effect on breast tissue density, an indicator of cancer risk.

More on Soy

Some people don't eat soy because they're just not familiar with it. The soybean is a member of the pea (legume) family. It forms clusters of three to five pods, each with two to four beans. Tofu, miso, tempeh and other foods made from soy contain isoflavones. Some soy products such as soy sauce and soy oil contain soy but are not good sources of isoflavones.

The Soyfoods Association of North America's website, SoyFoods.org, has descriptions of soy foods and recipes. *Example...*

THAI TOFU KEBABS

⅓ cup fresh lime juice (about 2 limes)
1 Tablespoon soy sauce

1 garlic clove, chopped
2 Tablespoons chopped Thai or Italian basil
½ tsp hot red pepper flakes
¼ tsp freshly ground black pepper
¼ cup olive oil
1 pound firm or extra firm tofu in one block
4-inch piece of cucumber, peeled
1 medium red onion, halved vertically and cut into half-inch crescents
8 cherry tomatoes

To make the marinade, combine the lime juice, soy sauce, garlic, basil, red pepper flakes, black pepper and olive oil in a resealable plastic bag. Cut the pressed tofu into 12 cubes. Add the tofu to the bag. Marinate in the refrigerator for at least four hours and up to 24 hours.

Soak four 10-inch bamboo skewers in water for 15 to 30 minutes. Preheat a grill to medium-high or a broiler.

Halve the cucumber lengthwise. Scoop out the seeds with a teaspoon. Cut each piece into one-inch crescents.

To assemble, slip a cucumber piece almost to the bottom of a skewer. Add a tofu chunk. Slip on two or three onion crescents, followed by a tomato. Repeat.

Grill or broil kebabs for two minutes. Brush them with some marinade. Cook another minute. Turn and cook two to three minutes, until the tofu is hot and the vegetables lightly charred, brushing them with marinade halfway through. Serves four.

Best Foods for Your Skin

Torey Armul, MS, RD, CSSD, LD, is a registered dietitian, nutritionist and national media spokesperson for the Academy of Nutrition and Dietetics. She is author of *Bun Appétit: A Simple Guide to Eating Right During Pregnancy.* Armul provides private counseling and consulting services in Columbus, Ohio.

Want healthier skin and fewer wrinkles? Men and women can look younger and lower their risk for skin cancer, psoriasis, eczema and more by eating certain foods. *The following foods have been scientifically proven to boost the health, strength and appearance of your skin...*

Yellow Bell Peppers

Yellow bell peppers are one of the most abundant sources of vitamin C. The body depends on vitamin C to form collagen, a protein that provides strength, support and elasticity to skin, hair, muscles and other tissues. Collagen also assists with cell regrowth and repair. As we age, our bodies produce less collagen, which can lead to reduced elasticity of the skin and more wrinkles.

The relationship between vitamin C and skin appearance was studied in more than 4,000 women in a report published in *The American Journal of Clinical Nutrition*. Researchers found that higher dietary intake of vitamin C was associated with lower likelihood of skin dryness and fewer wrinkles, as assessed by dermatologists. These results were independent of age, race, sun exposure, body mass index and physical activity.

Why not eat oranges, famous for their vitamin C, instead? A typical large orange contains 163% of the recommended daily value (DV) of vitamin C. That's good—but just half a yellow bell pepper contains nearly 300% of the DV of vitamin C. (Red and green peppers have less vitamin C than yellow ones but still are excellent sources.)

Eat yellow peppers raw to maximize the nutrient content. Vitamin C is sensitive to cooking and, as a water-soluble vitamin, leaches into cooking water. If you prefer to cook yellow peppers, keep the heat as low as possible for your recipe. Use the cooking juices, too (whenever possible), so that the vitamin C in the water is not wasted.

Sweet Potatoes

Sweet potatoes are an excellent source of carotenoids, the antioxidant pigments that give many foods their bright red, orange, yellow and green colors—and help keep skin cells healthy.

In a study published in *British Journal of Nutrition*, participants who ate more carotenoid-rich vegetables had significantly fewer facial wrinkles.

Eating carotenoids also can make you look healthier overall and more attractive to others. Carotenoid levels in skin contribute to healthy skin coloration. In fact, researchers from University of St. Andrews, Scotland, found that people whose faces were rated as healthy by others had consumed an average of 2.9 fruit and vegetable portions each day...and whose faces were rated separately as attractive had consumed 3.3 daily portions.

Carotenoids are fat-soluble, which means that they're better absorbed when paired with a fat-containing food—so sprinkle nuts or drizzle olive oil over your sweet potatoes for a delicious skin boost.

Salmon

Although protein in your food does not directly affect protein in your body's collagen, some research shows that amino acids (the building blocks of protein) are related to collagen synthesis in the skin.

Some amino acids are "essential," meaning that they're necessary for life but are not made in the body. They must be provided by food or supplements. Salmon contains all the essential amino acids—and essential amino acids play a unique role in skin health. In a study published in *Amino Acids*, researchers found that consuming a combination of essential amino acids significantly increased the rate of collagen synthesis in mice with UV-damaged skin.

Salmon also is a good source of monounsaturated fat, which was found to be positively associated with skin elasticity in older women in a study published in *British Journal of Nutrition*.

Don't love fish? Essential amino acids also are found in poultry, eggs, beans and whole grains.

Walnuts

Walnuts are rich in omega-3 polyunsaturated fatty acids, which help the body make the collagen needed for healthy skin. Omega-3s help reduce inflammation and have been shown to reduce symptoms in inflammatory skin diseases such as psoriasis and acne.

The European Journal of Cancer published research comparing omega-3 fat intake to the development of malignant melanoma in more than 20,000 women. Data showed that higher intakes of omega-3s were associated with an 80% lower risk for skin cancer, leading researchers to conclude that these fats "have a substantial protective association" against melanoma.

Like essential amino acids, omega-3 fats are vitally important but are not made in the body. You must get them from your diet or supplements. Aside from walnuts (and salmon, discussed above), other excellent sources of omega-3s include flaxseed oil, ground flaxseed, chia seeds, canola oil and tofu.

Raspberries and Pomegranates

There is exciting research on collagen and how it is affected by ellagic acid, an antioxidant found in certain fruits and vegetables.

A study published in *Experimental Dermatology* found that mice who received ellagic acid had significantly reduced collagen breakdown from UV light, compared with mice who did not receive ellagic acid. The treatment group also developed fewer wrinkles. While most research focuses on the treatment of skin damage, this study was unique in its ability to show the role of nutrition in the prevention of collagen breakdown, wrinkles and skin damage.

Foods that are high in ellagic acid include raspberries and pomegranates (as well as blackberries, strawberries and cranberries).

Chickpeas

Zinc is an important ingredient for skin health because it supports the regeneration of new skin cells. The benefits are most apparent with skin repair and wound healing, but zinc also may be able to help with other skin problems such as rashes, eczema and acne.

A study published in *BioMed Research International* found a correlation between participants' zinc levels and the severity of their acne symptoms. Researchers believe that this is partly due to zinc's ability to inhibit the overgrowth of Propionibacterium acnes, a bacterium that contributes to acne.

Legumes were the focus of another study in *The Journal of the American College of Nutrition*. Researchers found that higher intakes of legumes, such as chickpeas, appeared to protect against sun-induced wrinkles in people with a variety of ethnic and geographic backgrounds.

Chickpeas are a good source of zinc, as are other beans, oysters, poultry, tofu, oatmeal and zinc-fortified cereals.

CHAPTER 14

Best Foods for Weight Management

Foods That Rev Up Your Metabolism

Ridha Arem, MD, an endocrinologist, director of the Texas Thyroid Institute, an endocrinologist practice at Texas Medical center in Houston. He is a former chief of endocrinology and metabolism at Houston's Ben Taub General Hospital and is author of *The Thyroid Solution Diet*. AremWellness.com

Forget about calories! Most people who are trying to lose weight worry too much about calories and not enough about the actual cause of those extra pounds.

The real culprit: Out-of-balance hormones.

Best approach for controlling weight: A diet that rebalances the body's hormones. Carefully chosen foods and food combinations rebalance levels and/or efficiency of metabolism-regulating hormones, such as ghrelin, leptin and thyroid hormone. You'll burn more calories, and your body will be less likely to store calories as fat. Here's how...

Tweaking the Best Diets

Hands down, the Mediterranean diet is one of the healthiest diets out there. With its emphasis on plant-based foods (such as vegetables, fruits, grains and nuts) and healthful fats (from fatty fish and olive oil), it is good for your heart and helps control blood sugar levels.

But for more efficient weight loss, you need to go a step further. That's where the Protein-Rich Oriental Diet, developed by Korean researchers, enters the picture. With its heavy focus on high-protein foods, this diet has been found to provide twice the weight loss offered by calorie restriction alone.

To achieve and maintain an optimal body weight: The diet I designed includes elements of both these diets—as well as some important additional tweaks such as timing your meals (see page 192) and consuming a mix of proteins in order to get the full complement of amino acids, which is essential for increasing metabolism and controlling hunger. On my diet, you will eat a combination of at least two proteins, good fats and vegetables at each meal. *For example...*

•**Fish, turkey and chicken contain all of the essential amino acids that are in red meat, but with fewer calories and less saturated fat.** They're particularly rich in arginine, an amino acid that increases the speed at which your body burns calories.

My advice: Aim for six to eight ounces of these foods as the primary protein for dinner. You also can include these foods at breakfast and lunch as one of your protein choices.

•**Reduced-fat cottage cheese, ricotta, yogurt and goat cheese.** Certain forms of dairy are high in branched-chain amino acids, which suppress appetite and increase the ability of mitochondria (the energy-producing components of cells) to burn fat.

My advice: Each day, eat about a half-cup of low-fat or nonfat dairy as a protein.

•**High-protein beans, lentils and grains, such as black beans, kidney beans, quinoa and brown rice.** Eat one of these protein sources (three-fourths cup to one cup) at lunch—usually combined with a small serving of fish or lean meat. In addition to packing plenty of protein and fiber, these foods provide large amounts of amino acids that will help you get fitter and have more energy.

•**Egg whites contain all of the amino acids that you need for efficient weight loss, and they are my favorite choice as a protein for breakfast.** An egg-white omelet with onions, mushrooms and other vegetables can be prepared in just a few minutes. Limit your intake of egg yolks due to their cholesterol.

Low-Glycemic Carbs

Carbohydrates that are digested quickly—mainly refined and processed foods such as juices, white rice and French fries—increase insulin and fat storage.

Carbohydrates with a lower glycemic score are absorbed more slowly and don't cause unhealthy changes in insulin or fat storage.

Good choices: Whole oats, chickpeas and fruit (see below) at breakfast and lunch, and vegetables at each meal.

More Fiber

The fiber in such foods as beans and vegetables reduces appetite and slows digestion, important for preventing insulin "spikes." Research shows that people of normal weight tend to eat significantly more fiber than those who are overweight or obese.

For efficient weight loss: Get 35 g of fiber daily.

Fruit is also a good source of fiber. Just be sure that you choose fresh fruit that's low in natural sugar (fructose).

Good choices: Raspberries, strawberries, papayas, apples and cranberries. Avoid fruit at dinner to make it the lowest glycemic meal.

Green Tea

Green tea is high in epigallocatechin gallate (EGCG), a substance that can decrease the accumulation of body fat. It also increases insulin sensitivity and improves an obesity-related condition known as metabolic syndrome. Drink a few cups every day. Do not sweeten the tea with honey or other sweeteners—they are among the main causes of high insulin and weight gain.

Fish Oil Supplements

The omega-3 fatty acids in fish increase the rate at which calories are burned. However, even if you eat fish every day, it doesn't contain enough omega-3s for long-term weight control.

Solution: Take a daily supplement with 600 mg of EPA and 400 mg of DHA—the main types of omega-3s. Check first with your doctor if you take blood thinners or diabetes medication, since fish oil may interact with these drugs.

Not Just for Weight Loss

A hormone-balancing eating plan can rev up your metabolism even if you don't need to lose weight, giving you more energy and mental focus. If you aren't overweight and you follow this eating plan, you may lose a pound or two, but mostly you'll just feel better.

Timing Matters!

When you eat is almost as important as what you eat...

•**Plan on eating four or five daily meals**—breakfast between 6 am and 8 am...an optional (and light) late-morning snack...lunch between 11 am and 12:30 pm...a mid-afternoon snack...and supper between 5 pm and 7 pm.

•**Plan your meals so that you get more protein at supper.** It will stimulate the release of growth hormone, which burns fat while you sleep.

•**Avoid all food three hours before bedtime.** Eating late in the evening causes increases in blood sugar and insulin that can lead to weight gain—even if you consume a lower-calorie diet (1,200 to 1,500 calories a day).

Food Swaps—All the Pleasure... None of the Guilt

Dawn Jackson Blatner, RD, a registered dietitian in private practice in Chicago. She is the author of *The Flexitarian Diet: The Mostly Vegetarian Way to Lose Weight, Be Healthier, Prevent Disease, and Add Years to Your Life*. She is also the nutrition consultant for the Chicago Cubs and writes a food and nutrition blog for *The Huffington Post*. Dawn JacksonBlatner.com

The next time you're craving a less-than-healthful treat, such as a plate of pasta or a bowl of ice cream, don't assume that it's off-limits.

There are plenty of good-for-you cooking and baking swaps that don't significantly alter the food's flavor and texture but will up the nutritional ante and save you calories. *My favorites...*

WHAT TO SKIP: **Bread crumbs.**

Try instead: Seeds.

Good choices: Sesame seeds, chopped pumpkin seeds or chopped sunflower seeds.

Most bread crumbs are nothing more than refined white bread. Coating fish or chicken with seeds delivers more flavor and a satisfying crunch along with healthful types of fat, satiating fiber and protein.

What to do: Sprinkle the seeds on a plate, and dip your fish or chicken in to coat it.

WHAT TO SKIP: Butter.

Try instead: Avocado.

When baking, you can substitute some—but not all—of the butter with puréed avocado. Try a ratio of 70% butter to 30% avocado at first. If the taste and texture are good, work toward a half-and-half mixture. Avocado has the same creamy texture as artery-clogging butter, but one tablespoon of avocado purée has far fewer calories (23 versus 100 calories) and is a good source of heart-healthy fat and fiber, cancer-fighting folate and blood pressure–regulating potassium.

WHAT TO SKIP: Pasta.

Try instead: Spaghetti squash.

A typical plate of pasta (about three cups) can easily cost you 600 calories, and that's before topping it with butter, oil or sauce. One cup (a more appropriate serving size) of spaghetti squash "pasta" has just 42 calories plus fiber and 9% of your daily requirement of vitamin C.

What to do: Slice a spaghetti squash in half, remove the seeds and place flesh side down on a baking sheet with a little water in it. Bake at 375°F for 40 minutes. Remove it from the oven, then with an oven mitt still on to protect your hands from the hot squash, run a fork through the flesh lengthwise—it will naturally separate into pastalike strands. Top it with a marinara sauce and lean ground turkey or chicken.

WHAT TO SKIP: Sour cream.

Try instead: Greek yogurt.

Greek yogurt is essentially yogurt that has been strained to remove much of the liquid and sugar. It has twice as much protein as regular yogurt (for almost the same amount of calories) and less than half as much sugar as regular yogurt. In fact, a six-ounce cup of nonfat Greek yogurt packs in 18 g of protein—almost as much as a small chicken breast! Greek yogurt has a similar look, taste and consistency to sour cream, which is typically high in saturated fat and low in protein.

WHAT TO SKIP: White or brown rice.

Try instead: Cauliflower "rice."

One cup of medium-grain white rice contains 242 calories with very little fiber (brown rice has 218 calories). The same amount of cauliflower has only 14 calories, plus 22% of your daily need for vitamin K, which helps with blood clotting and bone health. As a cruciferous vegetable, cauliflower is thought to help protect against cancer of the mouth, pharynx, larynx, esophagus and stomach.

To make cauliflower "rice": Pulse fresh, raw cauliflower in a food processor until it resembles rice grains. Briefly steam or sauté it.

WHAT TO SKIP: Cream cheese.

Try instead: Puréed cottage cheese.

One tablespoon of cream cheese contains 50 calories and 3 g of saturated fat. For a leaner, higher protein bagel spread or to use on sliced veggies or fruit, try puréeing 1% or 2% milk fat cottage cheese in a blender. It will have a look and consistency that's similar to cream cheese but a slightly saltier flavor. Play up the savory aspect by adding chopped chives, basil and parsley—or go sweeter with a sprinkle of cinnamon. To save on time and effort, use pre-whipped cottage cheese.

WHAT TO SKIP: Ice cream.

Try instead: Frozen banana soft serve.

Frozen bananas, when blended at a high speed, achieve a creamy, ice cream–like consistency.

What to do: Chop a ripe banana into small pieces and freeze in a plastic bag (spread pieces out flat to avoid a large frozen clump.) The colder the bananas are, the thicker the dessert. Toss frozen pieces in a blender, and add a splash of low-fat milk. Start the blender on low, then do high pulses until the mixture is thick and creamy.

You'll save hundreds of calories (a medium banana has 105 calories…a cup of premium ice cream has 369), plus it's fat-free and rich in potassium and vitamins C and B-6. Toss in antioxidant-rich blueberries. Or sprinkle with cinnamon—it helps stabilize blood sugar…unsweetened cocoa powder, which is low-calorie…or chopped walnuts for a dose of heart-friendly fats.

Why Creamy Peanut Butter Is Fattening…It's Not the Fat

Study of effects of carboxymethylcellulose and polysorbate-80 on human gut bacteria by Benoit Chassaing, PhD, assistant professor of biomedical sciences, and colleagues, Georgia State University, Atlanta, presented at 2016 Digestive Disease Week in San Diego.

Would you want to eat "soapy" food? Well, you might be doing that if you eat peanut butter, ice cream, sherbet, mayonnaise, salad dressing, icing, pudding, candy, cottage cheese or cream cheese.

Depending on how they are manufactured, each of these foods may contain actual detergent.

It's in many everyday foods, and besides being disgusting to think about eating, it could be setting the stage for digestive ills, cardiovascular troubles and weight gain.

Messing with the Gut

There's growing evidence that certain particular ingredients in many processed foods may interfere with digestion, setting the stage for digestive illnesses, cardiovascular risk and weight gain. They're called emulsifiers—a kind of detergent that's added to improve texture and prolong shelf life. When food manufacturers remove fat from foods, they often add emulsifiers to create a smoother product.

The latest evidence: Two of the most common emulsifiers in our food supply—carboxymethylcellulose and polysorbate-80—can alter beneficial gut bacteria in nasty ways. We already reported on an earlier study that found that these compounds change the mucous membrane of the gut so that healthy bacteria leak out, triggering inflammation. This inflammation starts a chain reaction that could lead to diseases such as ulcerative colitis, Crohn's disease and inflammatory bowel disease—as well as metabolic syndrome, which can lead to diabetes and heart disease.

In a follow-up study, the same researchers at Georgia State University have found that the damage begins even before bacteria leak out of the gut. Using lab equipment that simulates the human gut, researchers added the two emulsifiers to the human gut bacteria. Markers for inflammation increased significantly.

The researchers then implanted the altered gut bacteria into gut-bacteria–free mice. Result: The mice developed intestinal inflammation and showed signs of metabolic syndrome.

What to Do Now

It's still early research, to be sure—human studies are planned—and there's no way to know yet how important a role these ingredients actually play in these common diseases.

It's not known whether other emulsifiers have similar negative effects. However, carrageenan, a gum that is also commonly used as an emulsifier, has been linked in other animal studies to gut inflammation.

But the research is enough to make us read labels pretty carefully—at least for a start. *For instance, these two additives, which are labeled as safe for food by the FDA, go by a variety of names...*

•**Carboxymethylcellulose** is also known as cellulose gum, carboxymethyl cellulose, sodium carboxymethyl cellulose, CMC, modified cellulose and cellulose gel.

•**Polysorbate 80** is also known as polyoxythylene sorbitan mono-oleate and Tween 80.

However, even careful label reading can only take you so far, since possible gut-harming emulsifiers lurk in many processed foods. The easiest way to play it safe? Choose minimally processed foods that contain only ingredients you recognize. You can find ice cream that contains just cream, milk and sugar, for example. And when it comes to peanut butter, whether smooth or crunchy, look for those that contain just peanuts, or peanuts and salt.

CHAPTER 15

How to Eat and Cook For Better Health

Easy Cooking Tricks for Much Healthier Foods

Lisa R. Young, PhD, RD, CDN, a nutritionist in private practice and an adjunct professor in the department of nutrition and food studies at New York University in New York City. She is the author of *The Portion Teller Plan: The No-Diet Reality Guide to Eating, Cheating, and Losing Weight Permanently.*

Loading up your grocery cart with fruits and vegetables is a great start to a healthful diet. But even if you hit the produce section on a regular basis, chances are you're not getting the same level of nutrients in your fruits and vegetables that earlier generations did.

Modern agricultural methods have stripped soil of important nutrients, so produce that is eaten today may be less healthful than it used to be.*

Troubling findings: A study published in the *Journal of the American College of Nutrition* found "reliable declines" in the amount of key vitamins and minerals in 43 fruits and vegetables compared with nutrient levels of those foods in 1950.

Other research has found that the levels of calcium in 12 fresh veggies dropped, on average, by 27%...iron by 37%...and vitamin C by 30% over a 22-year period. Such changes in nutrient values can have a hidden danger by contributing to nutrition deficiencies, which are more common than one might imagine finding in the US.

*Organic fruits and vegetables may have more nutrients than those that are conventionally grown.

For these reasons, it's crucial for you to do everything you can to squeeze all of the available nutrition from your foods. Besides stocking up on fruits and veggies, studies have shown that how you store, prepare and cook foods—and even how you combine them—can make a difference. *Six tricks that will help you get the greatest nutrition from your foods…*

• **Make steaming your first choice.** Vegetables are good for you no matter how they're prepared. But to get the most nutrients, steaming is the best choice.

Scientific evidence: Steamed broccoli retained virtually all the tested antioxidants in a study published in the *Journal of the Science of Food and Agriculture*, while microwaved broccoli lost 74% to 97% of these disease-fighting nutrients—possibly because microwaves can generate higher temperatures than other cooking methods.

Boiling is also problematic. The liquid—combined with the high heat and lengthy cooking time—strips out significant levels of important nutrients.

Example: Broccoli that's been boiled loses large amounts of glucosinolate, a compound that's been linked to cancer prevention.

Helpful: The liquid does retain nutrients, so consider using it in a soup.

A caveat: If you simply don't have time to steam your veggies and, as a result, risk not eating them, microwaving can be an acceptable option—if you add only a teaspoon or so of water and cook for the shortest time possible to retain nutrients.

Even though microwaving has been found to remove certain nutrients, it can be one of the best ways to preserve vitamin C and other water-soluble nutrients because the cooking times tend to be shorter. Other methods, such as sautéing and roasting, retain nutrients if you don't cook vegetables at high temperatures or for too long.

• **Cooked beats fresh.** Fresh, minimally processed foods should usually be your first choice—but not with tomatoes. Cooked tomatoes or canned tomato sauce or paste (best in a BPA-free can or glass jar) provides more lycopene than fresh tomatoes. Lycopene is a well-studied antioxidant that's been linked to reduced risk for prostate and other cancers, along with reduced risk for stroke.

Scientific evidence: A study in *The American Journal of Clinical Nutrition* found that the lycopene in tomato paste has 2.5 times the bioavailability of the lycopene in fresh tomatoes.

Why: The heat used during processing breaks down cell walls and releases more of the compound. Also, the oils that are added to processed tomatoes make it easier for the body to absorb lycopene.

•**Cook first, chop later.** Many people chop their veggies first, then add them to dishes before they go on the stove or into the oven.

Smart idea: Chop most veggies after you've done the cooking.

Here's why: Vitamin C and other nutrients oxidize when they're exposed to air for an extended period of time. An oxidized vitamin loses some of its bioactivity. In addition, chopped or diced vegetables have a greater surface area than whole ones, which allows more nutrients to leach into cooking liquids.

Exception: Onions and garlic should be chopped first (see page 200).

Scientific evidence: A recent study found that carrots, chopped before cooking, had 25% less falcarinol, a natural anticancer compound, than cooked whole carrots.

•**Try lemon (or lime) to boost iron levels.** Iron deficiency is among the most common nutrition deficiencies in the US, particularly among women of childbearing age. Meats are high in iron, but women with heavy periods might need more.

Low iron can also be a problem for vegetarians/vegans. That's because the non-heme iron in plant foods isn't as readily absorbed as the heme iron in meats.

Helpful: Add a little vitamin C–rich lemon or lime juice to recipes. Research shows that vitamin C can boost the absorption of non-heme iron by fourfold.

•**Add a spoonful of fat.** A garden-fresh salad or a plate of steamed broccoli is undoubtedly healthy. But for an even greater nutrient boost, add a teaspoon of olive oil.

You need fat to absorb vitamin E, beta-carotene, vitamin A and other fat-soluble nutrients/antioxidants. The average meal contains more than enough fat to get the job done, but simpler, fat-free meals won't provide that extra boost.

Healthier Grilling

Grilling meat, poultry and fish at high temperatures can lead to the formation of two types of potential carcinogens, polycyclic aromatic hydrocarbons (PAH) and heterocyclic amines (HCA).

A healthier option: Create your meal with grilled vegetables and fruit. Because they require a lot less grill time, fewer PAHs are formed. Cut veggies, such as portobello mushrooms, eggplant or zucchini, into chunks for kabobs, cook in a grill basket or grill whole. Brush with olive oil or marinade to prevent sticking. Choose fruit that is a day away from being ripe so that it will hold up on the grill. Watch closely, as fruit and veggies generally cook quickly. Try apples, pineapples or peaches.

Alice Bender, RDN, head of nutrition programs, American Institute for Cancer Research, Washington, DC.

My advice: Add a little bit of olive oil to dishes…or dress up fat-free dishes with ingredients that contain healthy fats, such as nuts, olives, feta cheese or a hard-boiled egg.

•**Chop garlic, and let it sit.** Many people love the robust flavor of whole garlic cloves that are roasted to buttery smoothness. But you'll get more health benefits from garlic that's been chopped.

Garlic (as well as onions) contains allicin and other sulfur-containing compounds that are locked within cell walls. The cells rupture when these foods are minced or chopped (or well-chewed), which releases enzymes that transform alliin into allicin, a compound with cardiovascular and anticancer benefits.

Good rule of thumb: Chopping and letting garlic or onions sit for about 10 minutes will allow the enzyme to make the healthful conversion. Heating garlic or onions before the completion of the enzymatic reaction will reduce the health benefits.

Good-for-You Comfort Food

Laura Cipullo, RD, CDE, a registered dietitian and certified diabetes educator in private practice in New York City. Cipullo is author of *The Diabetes Comfort Food Diet* and is president of the New York chapter of the International Association of Eating Disorders Professionals.

As a health-conscious reader, you probably know that limiting carb intake while increasing fiber and reducing saturated fat is a healthful eating plan to follow. But you're human, and it can be oh, so hard to resist carbohydrate-laden, high-calorie comfort foods like creamy mashed potatoes and rich pasta dishes.

Good news: With a few smart tweaks and swaps, you can enjoy even the most decadent-sounding comfort foods without sabotaging your health. *Here's how…**

•**Get the right amount of carbohydrates.** You don't need to eliminate carbs entirely, you just need to eat the right amount, which is probably more than you think.

*Note: The recipes in this article were developed for people with diabetes, but those who don't have diabetes and people with other conditions can benefit as well.

Research shows that even people with diabetes who eat small, consistent amounts of carbohydrates with every meal or snack as opposed to eating excessive carbs at each meal or eating them once a day have better control of their blood sugar levels and body weight. However, the average woman who has prediabetes or diabetes should moderate carb intake to about 45 g per meal and men should have no more than about 60 g per meal. (A health-care provider can help adjust amounts based on individual needs.) The allowance is more generous for those who don't have diabetes, but everyone can benefit from sticking to these guidelines.

Some foods with 45 g of carbs: One cup of brown rice…one and a half English muffins. Not too stingy!

•**Fiber is your secret weapon.** Fiber—especially the soluble kind—takes longer to metabolize than other carbs, so it improves blood sugar control and lowers insulin resistance in both people who have diabetes and those who don't. Consistently getting the right amount of fiber can even lessen (or in some instances, eliminate) the need for diabetes medication. The American Diabetes Association recommends that women consume at least 25 g of fiber per day… men should get a minimum of 38 g daily. But aim for 44 g to 50 g a day to reap the health benefits above. Whole grains, beans, fruits and vegetables are all naturally high in fiber.

•**Don't forget healthy fats.** Replacing saturated fats and trans fats with monounsaturated fatty acids (MUFAs), such as olive oil, canola oil, peanut oil, nuts, nut butters and avocado, helps lower total and LDL "bad" cholesterol levels, improves the function of blood vessels and benefits insulin levels and blood sugar control.

The following are healthful comfort foods that meet the goals above…

CREAMY MASHED POTATOES

Instead of mashed potatoes loaded with saturated fat from butter, enjoy these mashed potatoes made with yogurt and a surprise ingredient…

What to do: In a large pot, combine 1 pound of peeled (I like to leave the peels on for extra fiber and nutrients) and halved russet (baking) potatoes and 1 small head of cauliflower, cut into florets. Cover with water, bring to a boil, then reduce heat to medium and simmer for 20 minutes, or until the potatoes and cauliflower are easily pierced with a fork. Drain and place in a large bowl with ⅓ cup of vegetable broth and 2 tablespoons of olive oil. Using an electric mixer on medium speed, beat until creamy. Add ½ cup of plain nonfat Greek yogurt and beat until just blended. Try adding garlic or rosemary if you desire. Makes six servings.

Traditional recipe: 250 calories per serving, 5 g saturated fat, 2 g fiber, 39 g carbs.

New recipe above: 132 calories, 1 g saturated fat, 3 g fiber, 19 g carbs.

Why it's good for you: The addition of cauliflower is a sneaky-but-healthy nutrition hack—cauliflower delivers more fiber than potatoes, while cutting the carb content of this dish in half! Plus, a 2014 study in *BMJ* offered further proof that diets high in produce are associated with lower risk for death, particularly cardiovascular mortality. Olive oil is a great source of MUFAs, and the yogurt adds creaminess and even a little protein while curbing carbs.

BROCCOLI PENNE

Instead of white, blood sugar–spiking pasta with high-fat alfredo sauce, have this healthful broccoli pasta dish with mozzarella...

What to do: Cook 6 ounces of multigrain penne pasta in boiling water. Add 2 cups of fresh broccoli florets to the pot during the last two minutes of cooking. Drain the pasta and broccoli, reserving ½ cup of the water. In a large bowl, place the pasta, broccoli, 1 cup of halved grape tomatoes, 6 ounces of fresh, part-skim mozzarella cheese cubed, ¼ cup of pesto sauce and 1 tablespoon of lemon juice. Add the reserved pasta water to the bowl, one tablespoon at a time, stirring gently until the ingredients are combined. Makes four servings.

Tip: Cook the pasta al dente (just until firm). Longer cooking times break down starches, which causes more carbohydrates to be absorbed into your blood, resulting in a faster rise in blood sugar.

Traditional recipe: 800 calories per serving, 30 g saturated fat, 4 g fiber, 69 g carbs.

New recipe above: 341 calories, 5 g saturated fat, 5 g fiber, 34 g carbs.

Why it's good for you: A 2015 study confirmed what we already knew—diets rich in whole grains protect against diabetes, while diets rich in refined carbohydrates like conventional white pasta increase risk. High-fiber broccoli and tomatoes fill you up, which enables you to halve the amount of pasta in this recipe. Flavorful olive oil–based pesto means you can pass on the alfredo sauce—full of artery-clogging saturated fat—and get a dose of MUFAs instead. (*Surprising:* Multigrain pasta contains MUFAs, too.) Ideally, make your own pesto using fresh basil, Parmesan cheese, olive oil, crushed garlic and pine nuts. If you're using store-bought pesto, choose a local brand, which is more likely to have high-quality ingredients and fewer preservatives than a big-box brand. Grilled chicken or trout goes well with this pasta dish.

The Most Powerful Food Secret—Some Healthy Foods Are Not Healthy When You Eat Them Together

Donna Gates, a nutritional consultant and lecturer and author of the best-selling book *The Body Ecology Diet: Rediscovering Your Health and Rebuilding Your Immunity.* She worked with Leonard Smith, MD, medical adviser for the University of Miami's department of integrative medicine, on *The Baby Boomer Diet: Body Ecology's Guide to Growing Younger.* Bodyecology.com

When I was 15, my skin began to break out, and a well-meaning but misguided dermatologist prescribed antibiotics. Fifteen years later, frequent use of antibiotics had weakened my body to the point where I had almost no functional immune system—and my stomach burned whenever I ate anything. By the time I was 30, I could tolerate only five foods.

For the next decade, I explored every kind of diet available, as well as many other natural-healing methods. Then I discovered that I had the systemic infection candidiasis, which had compromised my digestive, immune and endocrine systems. One tool I used to heal myself was food combining, a revolutionary approach to eating that I learned about in my research. I then worked with Leonard Smith, MD, medical adviser for the University of Miami's department of integrative medicine, to understand the science behind it.

Food combining focuses on the way you combine foods at each meal—the animal and vegetable proteins...the fats and oils...the starches...and the fruits and vegetables.

Some food combinations are easy to digest. They are quickly broken down, and the nutrients are thoroughly assimilated. Other combinations can be a digestive disaster, producing gas, bloating and other gastrointestinal (GI) discomforts.

Many Benefits

Proper food combining may mean that you no longer need to take medications for digestive problems. Food combining also has benefits for your overall health. *Here are the benefits you can expect...*

•**Less bloating, stomach pain and gas,** because well-digested foods don't ferment in the intestines, producing those symptoms.

•**Less heartburn,** because digestion is more efficient.

•**Better absorption of nutrients** and, therefore, a better-nourished body and more effective immune system.

•**Younger looks,** because poorly digested foods generate toxins that contribute to a dull complexion and a bloated body.

•**Weight control,** because properly combined foods are assimilated and metabolized better, reducing the likelihood that they will be stored as fat.

Six Simple Rules

The simple rules for food combining might not seem so simple at first. Don't expect to master them in a day.

My suggestion: Place the food-combining chart below on your refrigerator door. Or you can print out a copy at BodyEcology.com/foodcombiningchart. Then try food combining for a little while—even just three or four days. If you have digestive ills, you likely will find the benefits are immediate—gas, bloating and stomachaches will vanish.

RULE #1: **Eat animal protein with nonstarchy vegetables.** When you eat animal-protein foods (eggs, fish, poultry, red meat) with a starchy vegetable or grain (examples include artichokes, carrots, corn, oats, peas, potatoes, rice, wheat, winter squash and yams), your salivary glands secrete ptyalin and amylase that break down the grains and starchy vegetables into simple sugars. Coating your protein foods with sugars creates compounds called advanced glycation end products (AGEs). AGEs are linked to inflammation and immune reactions that can lead to diseases such as diabetes and cardiovascular disease. When eaten together, animal-protein and starchy foods also are much more difficult to digest.

Instead, eat animal protein with nonstarchy vegetables such as asparagus, broccoli, cabbage, cauliflower, celery, cucumber, garlic, green beans, leafy greens (such as kale and collards), onions, sea vegetables (such as wakame and dulse) and zucchini.

Good combination: Fish with stir-fried nonstarchy vegetables.

Combinations to avoid: Chicken and rice. Pasta with meat sauce.

RULE #2: Eat grains and grainlike seeds (amaranth, buckwheat, millet and quinoa) with starchy and/or nonstarchy vegetables. This combination is the easiest of all meals to digest. I prefer grainlike seeds over grains because they are gluten-free and higher in protein.

Good combinations: Brown rice stir-fried with onions, garlic, broccoli, yellow squash and red pepper. A potato, onion and quinoa sauté, with a leafy green salad.

Combinations to avoid: Beef hamburger on a wheat bun. Pizza with pepperoni.

RULE #3: Consume fruit and fruit juices alone and at least 30 minutes before any meal...or combined with a protein-fat (avocados, dairy products, nuts and seeds). Or eat acidic fruit combined with leafy green salads. Fruit and fruit juices pass through the digestive tract very quickly. When they are consumed with slower-digesting animal-protein foods, starchy vegetables or grains, they become trapped in the digestive tract with those foods and cause fermentation. You quickly experience bloating and gas.

Protein-fats combine well with acidic fruits. In food combining, acidic fruits include citrus fruits and juice, berries, cherries and pineapples.

Good combinations: Blueberries in yogurt with walnuts. Grapefruit with avocado on lettuce. Tomato in a leafy green salad.

Combinations to avoid: Traditional breakfast of eggs, orange juice and toast. Strawberries on top of cereal.

RULE #4: Combine fats and oils with any food. Nature created fats in such a way that they go with just about everything we eat.

Good combinations: Salmon in a leafy green salad with an extra-virgin olive oil dressing. Baked potato or acorn squash with butter. Quinoa tabouli salad with an extra-virgin olive oil dressing.

RULE #5: Combine protein-fats with protein-fats. Protein-fats are easily digested when eaten together.

Good combinations: Leafy greens with grated cheese, chopped walnuts and a dressing made with yogurt. A smoothie made in a blender with cucumber, celery, zucchini, yogurt, almonds and avocado.

Combinations to avoid: Grilled cheese sandwich. Yogurt with cereal.

RULE #6: **Combine beans with nonstarchy vegetables.** Beans are a protein-starch (a food that is predominantly starchy but also has naturally occurring protein), and because protein and starches don't combine well together, beans are difficult to digest, producing a lot of gas. Combining them with easily digested foods such as nonstarchy vegetables works best.

Good combinations: Black beans with onions, garlic, celery and kale. Garbanzo beans in a leafy green salad.

Combination to avoid: Beans and rice.

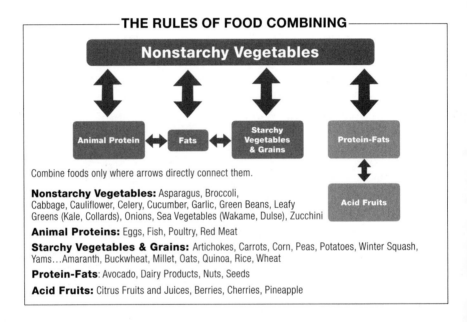

THE RULES OF FOOD COMBINING

Nonstarchy Vegetables

Animal Protein ⟷ Fats ⟷ Starchy Vegetables & Grains   Protein-Fats

Acid Fruits

Combine foods only where arrows directly connect them.

Nonstarchy Vegetables: Asparagus, Broccoli, Cabbage, Cauliflower, Celery, Cucumber, Garlic, Green Beans, Leafy Greens (Kale, Collards), Onions, Sea Vegetables (Wakame, Dulse), Zucchini

Animal Proteins: Eggs, Fish, Poultry, Red Meat

Starchy Vegetables & Grains: Artichokes, Carrots, Corn, Peas, Potatoes, Winter Squash, Yams...Amaranth, Buckwheat, Millet, Oats, Quinoa, Rice, Wheat

Protein-Fats: Avocado, Dairy Products, Nuts, Seeds

Acid Fruits: Citrus Fruits and Juices, Berries, Cherries, Pineapple

To Lose Weight, Cut Carbs...
Just Twice a Week

Louis Aronne, MD, professor of medicine, Weill Cornell Medical College, director, Comprehensive Weight Control Center at Weill Cornell Medicine and New York-Presbyterian, both in New York City.

There are many popular ways to lose weight. Lots of people try cutting calories across the board, but then they are hungry a lot of the time. Others dramatically cut carbs, which often helps with hunger, but that is hard to stick with if you love "carb-y" foods. Some people practice intermittent fasting, eating only 500 or 600 calories on certain days, but you might find that overly restrictive, too.

Fortunately, there is another, little-known approach that's just as effective as any of the above—and a whole lot easier for many people to stick with. Like intermittent fasting, it involves restrictive days, and like low-carb dieting, it involves drastically cutting carbohydrates. But here's the big difference: All you do is go low-carb twice a week, without counting calories at all. The rest of the week you eat as much of a normal healthy diet as you want. It may work by "resetting" the brain so that you're not as hungry—not just on low-carb days but even when you go back to your "normal" way of eating the rest of the week.

Here's how to make it work for you.

The Two-Day Low-Carb Diet

At the Comprehensive Weight Control Center at Weill Cornell Medical College, we became interested in this new approach when we reviewed a four-month British study of 115 overweight women. *The women were divided into three groups...*

Daily dieters cut their calories by 25% to an average of 1,500 a day on a balanced healthy Mediterranean-style diet.

A second group did intermittent fasting on two consecutive days. It was pretty intense—low-carb and no more than 600 calories a day...and then repeat the next day. The rest of the week, they ate as much as they wanted from a balanced diet.

The third group of women also went on an intermittent low-carb diet for two consecutive days, but they didn't have to restrict calories. It was a big carb reduction—to just 40 grams, slightly less than the amount in one cup of rice. On those days, they were allowed unrestricted protein and healthy fats. The rest of the week they ate as they wanted from a balanced diet.

Results: The two-day-a-week low-carb dieters lost just as much weight as the intermittent fasters...and lost more weight than the everyday dieters. And besides losing more weight (11 versus eight pounds), the two-day-a-weekers also lost more body fat, becoming lighter and leaner.

What was even more intriguing was that just cutting carbs on those two days—and not counting overall calories—was as effective as intermittent fasting. In fact, neither group tended to overeat on days when they weren't, respectively, cutting carbs or fasting.

Could it really be that easy to lose weight—just cut carbs two days a week? Yes, it could—because carbs do some very particular things to the brain.

The Carb-Brain-Appetite Connection

When you eat a lot of carbohydrates, especially simple starches and sugars, it can literally damage neurons in the hypothalamus, a part of the brain that helps regulate appetite. The nerve cells in the hypothalamus become surrounded by inflammatory cells, and then they don't function as well as they should.

Quality of fat matters, too. In animal studies, for example, high-saturated-fat diets—the kind of fats that are very prevalent in a typical Western diet—have also been shown to disrupt the appetite-signaling pathways. So the emphasis on healthy, mostly unsaturated fats in the diet may contribute to its effectiveness.

In effect, the brain becomes resistant to input from hormones, including leptin and ghrelin, which play key roles in regulating appetite. The hypothalamus mistakenly sends out signals to eat more. You feel hungrier, you eat more, and you create more damage—and so on.

The secret of the two-day-a-week carb-cutting diet is that the hunger-signaling pathway can be "reset" by giving the damaged neurons a break by cutting carbs, which also tends to cut calories, and by your eating healthy polyunsaturated and monounsaturated fats. When the oxidative load that's hitting those nerves decreases, the whole system can work much better.

That explains why people on this diet don't go crazy with overeating on their "off diet" days. Even after just one day of going very low carbohydrate, the signaling system between the appetite hormones and the hypothalamus works much more efficiently. That effect can last for a few days.

Ready to Try the Intermittent Low-Carb Diet?

In our clinical experience, we have found that there is no need to avoid carbohydrates two days in a row. We tell dieters that they are free to restrict their carbohydrates on any two days of the week.

For a lot of people, just eliminating bread, pasta and sweets (sugars are carbs) gets most of the job done. *But for a little more detail, here's a sample one-day low-carb menu...*

Breakfast: Two or three eggs with spinach and mozzarella cheese, made with one teaspoon of oil.

Lunch: A large vegetable salad with one-third of an avocado, five or more ounces of chicken or grilled shrimp or cheese, and one or two tablespoons of Italian dressing.

Snack: Six to eight ounces of Greek yogurt (0% to 2% fat) with eight walnut halves.

Dinner: Five or more ounces of grilled poultry, fish or red meat, roasted vegetables (such as cauliflower, Brussels sprouts or broccoli) with one or two tablespoons of olive oil, a tossed salad with one tablespoon of oil-and-vinegar and one cup of berries.

True, there's no linguine with clam sauce…no bread-and-jam. But it's only for a few days a week—and on the other five days, you may find that you're not craving carbs as much as you do now. You're almost sure to lose weight.

How to Eat Whole Grains on a Low-Carb Diet

Study titled "Whole grain consumption and risk of cardiovascular disease, cancer, and all cause and cause specific mortality: a systematic review and dose-response meta-analysis of prospective studies" by researchers at Imperial College of London, UK, published in *The BMJ*.

It's easy to feel confused about grains. On the one hand, you may be reducing your total carbs, which may mean cutting way back on pasta, rice, bread and other grain-based foods.

On the other hand, whole grains such as brown rice, whole wheat, oatmeal, buckwheat, whole-grain cornmeal and quinoa are not only nutritious but linked with protection against heart disease and other chronic ills.

So what's a health-conscious eater to do? What if you're watching your carbs—and your weight?

The good news, based on the latest research, is that you may need just a few servings of whole grains to get big health benefits. That fits nicely into a moderately low-carbohydrate diet.

The 90-gram Solution

To find out how much whole grain is associated with health benefits, an international team of public health researchers reported in *The BMJ* on a statistical meta-analysis of 45 studies from the US, Europe and Asia. Results…

Key finding: Eating just three servings of whole grains a day (90 grams) was statistically associated with a 16% reduced risk for cardiovascular disease, an 11% reduced risk for cancer and an 18% reduced risk for early death. (Eating whole grains was also linked with a lower risk for diabetes, respiratory illness and infectious disease, although specific optimal daily servings couldn't be calculated.)

•**People who ate just one or two servings of whole grains a day,** compared with those who ate none at all, were also protected from these chronic illnesses—and early death—in many studies.

•**Eating more than three servings (up to seven a day) was associated with a modest additional increase in benefit**—less heart disease, respiratory illness, cancer and early death in some studies.

•**Not surprisingly, people who ate more refined grains such as white bread received no health benefits.**

Why It's So Easy to Eat Enough Whole Grains

The other key point is that a serving is probably a lot less than you think. The researchers defined it as 30 grams of cooked food, which is about one ounce. The USDA defines a serving, based on one-ounce servings, as one small slice of bread...one-half cup of cooked brown rice...one-half cup of cooked whole-wheat pasta.

So eating just one small bowl of whole-grain cereal at breakfast (30 grams) and one large whole-wheat pita bread at dinner (60 grams) could easily bring you up to three servings for the day. Watch out for "portion distortion," too—a typical bagel, for example, can easily weigh in at four ounces (four servings) or more.

Bottom line: You can get most of the benefits of whole grains in your diet by aiming for three one-ounce (30-gram) servings a day.

Healthier Way to Cook Rice

Summary report of data on a study by researchers at the College of Chemical Sciences in Sri Lanka of how cooking methods affect resistant starch in rice, presented at the National Meeting and Exposition of the American Chemical Society in Denver.

Have you heard about the revolutionary new way to cook rice that cuts calories by as much as 60%? It's being touted online as a miracle weight-reducing kitchen trick, and it sounds like a dieter's dream.

Don't believe it. It isn't true.

But there is good science behind a rice-cooking technique that does cut calories—and makes rice less likely to spike your blood sugar levels.

Now that's healthy.

Rice Research

Researchers at the College of Chemical Sciences in Sri Lanka tested eight cooking variations on a variety of rice that's common in their country. One variation resulted in rice that had about 15% more resistant starch, a form of starch that our bodies can't digest, making it act more like fiber.

As a result, the rice cooked this way isn't likely to raise blood sugar as quickly as regular rice—a good thing, because rice, especially white rice, tends to send blood sugar up pretty quickly. Since resistant starch can't be digested, the new rice—at least the variety used in this study—also has about 10% to 15% fewer calories.

The 60% fewer calories claim? That came from the researchers speculating about what they might be able to achieve in future rice-cooking studies using other varieties of rice.

The Formula

The successful technique is pretty simple: Add about one teaspoon of coconut oil to each half cup of dry rice, cook normally—and then refrigerate it for 12 hours.

The best part: You don't have to eat the rice cold. You can enjoy it reheated and get the same benefits.

To Lower Breast Cancer Risk...

Longer gaps between the last food eaten in the evening and the first food eaten the next morning may reduce breast cancer risk. The longer the gap, the better the control over blood glucose concentrations—and this may lower risk for breast cancer. Each three-hour increase is associated with a 4% lower glucose level after eating, no matter how much food a woman consumes.

Study of dietary data for 2,212 women and glucose readings for 1,066 women by researchers in the cancer-prevention program, University of California, San Diego, published in *Cancer Epidemiology, Biomarkers & Prevention.*

The oil combines with the starch, and cooling the rice turns that starch into resistant starch. You could also use a different oil such as olive oil, although only coconut oil was used in this study. The cooling technique is well-known to food researchers—potatoes that are boiled then cooled tend to have more resistant starch, for example.

All in all, it's a pretty simple change that could have health benefits. Thinking of rice for tomorrow's dinner? You could cook up a batch tonight—and use it tomorrow. Any healthy recipe for leftover rice is a good place to start.

Eat This Plus That!

Tonia Reinhard, MS, RD, registered dietitian and professor at Wayne State University, Detroit. She is the program director for the Coordinated Program in Dietetics, co-director of clinical nutrition in the Wayne State University School of Medicine and past president of the Michigan Dietetic Association. She is author of *Superfoods: The Healthiest Foods on the Planet* and *Superjuicing: More Than 100 Nutritious Vegetable and Fruit Recipes.*

Well-chosen food pairings do more than just excite your taste buds. Consuming certain food combos or food and drink combos creates a synergy that increases the absorption of important nutrients and phytochemicals.

Here are four supercharged combinations…

Fish + Wine

The American Heart Association recommends eating fish at least twice a week. The omega-3 fatty acids in fish have been shown to reduce triglycerides, irregular heartbeats and blood pressure and slow the growth of arterial plaques. It turns out that wine can boost those omega-3 levels.

A large European study looked at the dietary habits and alcohol consumption of more than 1,600 people. The participants underwent comprehensive medical exams and gave blood samples that were used to measure omega-3 levels. Their amount of "marine food intake," defined as the total intake of fish, shellfish, cuttlefish, squid, octopus, shrimp and crab, was also measured.

The researchers found that people who drank moderate amounts of alcohol (one daily drink for women and two for men) had higher concentrations of omega-3s than nondrinkers, despite consuming similar amounts of marine food. Wine drinkers had the biggest gains, but people who drank beer or spirits (such as Scotch) also showed an increase in omega-3s.

Important caveat: The study found that heavy drinkers had lower amounts of omega-3s.

Lemon + Tea

Both black and green teas contain catechins, a group of antioxidants that are surprisingly good for cardiovascular health. A study published in *Stroke*, which looked at more than 83,000 Japanese adults, found that those who drank two to three cups of green tea daily were 14% less likely to have a stroke than those who rarely drank tea.

Tea has been found to reduce cholesterol and reduce the risk for cancer, diabetes and heart disease. But there's a catch—the catechins in tea aren't very durable. They tend to break down during digestion, leaving behind less than 20% of the active compounds.

Tasty solution: Add a squeeze of lemon to your tea. A laboratory study published in *Molecular Nutrition & Food Research* found that combining lemon juice with tea allowed 80% of the catechins to "survive" post-digestion. Orange, lime and grapefruit juices also stabilized the compounds, although not as much as the lemon.

If you prefer bottled to brewed tea, you'll get a similar effect by picking a product that includes vitamin C—listed as ascorbic acid on the label.

Citrus + Iron-Rich Foods

Low iron is common in people who take acid-suppressing drugs for GERD and in people who have gastrointestinal problems in which inflammation and bleeding occur (such as inflammatory bowel disease and bleeding ulcers).

Many foods contain iron. Iron-rich animal foods include beef, liver, oysters and sardines. Iron-rich plant foods include dark leafy greens such as spinach, kale and collard greens...beans...lentils...whole grains...and nuts. But iron is not the easiest mineral to absorb. The body can absorb only 2% to 20% of the non-heme iron in plant foods. The absorption of the heme iron from meats and fish/shellfish is better but still not great—typically between 15% and 35%. And certain supplements such as calcium can interfere with iron absorption.

How can you boost absorption of iron? By eating citrus fruits or other vitamin C–rich foods such as strawberries and yellow and red peppers with heme or non-heme foods. Examples: Add orange slices to your kale salad...or yellow peppers to your beef stew. One study found that consuming as little as 63 mg of vitamin C (a little more than the amount in one orange) nearly tripled the absorption of non-heme iron.

Fat + Salad

Salads are rich in carotenoids—antioxidants such as lutein, lycopene and beta-carotene that reduce your risk for cancer and heart disease, preserve bone density and prevent macular degeneration. A fat-based salad dressing can maximize the absorption of these carotenoids (so avoid fat-free salad dressings). Researchers at Purdue University served participants salads with dressings made from a monounsaturated fat (canola oil)...a polyunsaturated fat (soybean oil)...or a saturated fat (butter). All the fats boosted absorption of the carotenoids, but the monounsaturated fat required the least amount of fat to get the most carotenoid absorption. Another monounsaturated fat often found in salad dressings is olive oil.

You can get similar benefits by adding hard-boiled eggs to your salad. The fat from the yolks will increase your absorption of carotenoids. In a Purdue University study published in *The American Journal of Nutrition*, participants who ate a salad with one-and-a-half eggs had double the carotenoid absorption of people who had a salad with no eggs.

Five Healthy, Edible Weeds That Are Probably Growing in Your Yard

Mary Ellen Camire, PhD, president, Institute of Food Technologists, and professor of food science and human nutrition at the University of Maine, Orono...Chris Kilham, instructor of ethnobotany, University of Massachusetts, Amherst, and founder, Medicine Hunter, an enterprise that explores plant-based medicines.

You've plucked them and chucked them into your trash or compost pile. You've cursed their very existence. You've racked your brain trying to think of better ways to deal with the weeds in your yard—but have you ever considered eating them?

A Few Precautions

Before you even consider eating a weed that's growing wild, pay attention to these two safety rules...

•**Know your weeds.** There are many lookalikes in the plant kingdom. Of course, anyone can recognize a dandelion, but if you're not sure about a plant, don't eat it. To learn to identify what's edible and what's not in your region, look for a "wild foraging" workshop at your local Cooperative Extension, arboretum or chapter of the Audubon Society. You can also look up plants in books such as the classic *Stalking the Wild Asparagus* by Euell Gibbons or *Edible Wild Plants: A North American Field Guide to Over 200 Natural Foods* by Thomas Elias and Peter Dykeman...or check online resources, such as the West Virginia Department of Agriculture's publication, *Edible Wild Plants.*

•**Go organic—and beyond.** Pick weeds only from areas that haven't been treated with pesticides or herbicides, and avoid plants that have been exposed to high levels of car exhaust, such as those that grow alongside roads, near septic leach fields or businesses that use chemicals, or near any other potential sources of contamination. Even if the yard or field is organic and unpolluted, you'll want to rinse the plants thoroughly before you eat them to remove grit and insects. It's also not a good idea to collect food from any site where animal feces have contaminated the plants.

Ready? Here's how to safely enjoy five tasty, nutritious and even healing garden-variety weeds that grow plentifully throughout the country.

Supergreens and Healing Herbs

These common weeds are delicious...

•**Dandelion.** It's common, familiar—and eminently edible. The leaves have the best flavor—they're a little bitter, like broccoli rabe, and can be added raw to salads or sautéed. The stems and roots are less tasty but are fine if picked young and chopped and steamed or sautéed with other vegetables. Besides adding an earthy taste, fresh dandelion leaves provide a hefty dose of vitamin A, calcium, iron, vitamin E and potassium. You can also dry and roast the roots and then grind and brew them for a delicious coffeelike drink without caffeine.

•**Lambsquarters.** This weed has nothing to do with baby sheep—it's actually related to spinach. It grows throughout much of the US, especially in the summer months. A mild green that tastes a little like spinach, lambsquarters is often paired with mesclun (a leafy green) in restaurant salads, and it can also be steamed, sautéed or added to soups. It's a good source of fiber, calcium, magnesium and potassium, as well as vitamins A and C. A three-and-a-half-ounce serving (about a cup and a half), for example, provides 80 mg of vitamin

C—and a generous 300 mg of calcium. (Compare that to the same serving size of the "superfood" kale with a mere 135 mg of calcium!).

•**Fiddlehead ferns.** These little beauties are the furled fronds from a young ostrich fern, and they are hot items in farmers' markets and trendy restaurants these days, especially in the early spring. (*Note:* Make sure the fiddleheads you're collecting really are ostrich ferns and not bracken ferns, which are carcinogenic.) Fiddleheads should never be consumed raw or undercooked because of a risk for illness (the exact reason why some people get sick from eating them raw isn't known, but when you thoroughly cook them they're completely safe). Rinse them thoroughly, gently steam or boil, and then sauté them, perhaps with some olive oil, chopped garlic or onions, salt and pepper, Kilham suggests. Fiddleheads are nutritious as well as delicious, with a taste like earthy asparagus...a solid source of calcium, iron, magnesium, potassium, vitamins A and C, and niacin.

•**Elderberry.** The flowers and purple-blue berries of the elderberry plant are edible...the leaves are not. The berries can be made into jam, syrup, pies, even wine, while the large gossamer-like flower clusters can be dipped in pancake batter and pan-fried like a crepe. You can eat elderberries fresh off the bush or tossed into a salad for a hint of sweetness. With every cup of these berries, you'll get a substantial serving of fiber, calcium, iron, potassium and vitamin C. Elderberry syrup may boost the immune system, so it might help you skip your next cold or bout of flu. To make it, collect about one-half or three-quarters cup of berries, dry them, then boil them in three cups of water for a half hour or more, cool, strain, mix with one cup of honey and store in the refrigerator.

•**Red clover.** A wild perennial plant that belongs to the legume family, red clover is nutritious and may have medicinal properties. The leaves, which taste slightly like alfalfa sprouts, can be tossed into salads, sautéed or added to soups, and they are quite nutritious, containing calcium, magnesium, potassium, vitamin C, niacin and thiamine. But it's the weed's red flowers, which have a mildly sweet taste, that get the most attention. They are rich in isoflavones, compounds that act as estrogens, so it's not surprising that red clover tea is a common remedy for menopausal symptoms such as hot flashes. So far, study results are inconclusive, some finding a benefit and others not, but if you want to try it, dry the flowers, then steep a teaspoon or two in a cup of just-boiled water for a half an hour, and drink two or three cups a day.

Your Wild Edible Garden Awaits

Next time you fret about weeds in your yard or garden, remember that some of them are actually delicious plants that no one appreciates. Of course, now that you're acquainted with some of the tastier weeds, you may want to take the easier route and just look for them in your local farmers market. Chances are you'll find fiddleheads in the spring and big bunches of dandelion greens and lambsquarters all summer long and into the fall.

Good News About Frying Vegetables... in Olive Oil

Sharon Palmer, RDN, a registered dietitian and author of *The Plant-Powered Diet* and *Plant-Powered for Life*. She is the editor of *Environmental Nutrition* and nutrition editor of *Today's Dietician*. SharonPalmer.com

Study titled "Phenols and the antioxidant capacity of Mediterranean vegetables prepared with extra-virgin olive oil using different domestic cooking techniques" by researchers at the University of Granada, published in *Food Chemistry*.

Could frying vegetables in olive oil be the healthiest way to cook them? That's the suggestion of a recent Spanish study. It found that sautéing vegetables—even frying them—in extra-virgin olive oil resulted in dishes that were richer in certain health-promoting compounds than leaving them raw or boiling them.

But don't start frying all your veggies just yet. There's more to the story.

Why Olive Oil Should Touch Your Veggies When You Cook Them

In the study, researchers at the University of Granada in Spain looked at four vegetables commonly found in the Mediterranean diet—tomato, eggplant, pumpkin and potato. They cubed them and then cooked them different ways—boiled in water, boiled in water plus extra virgin olive oil (EVOO), sautéed in EVOO or fried in EVOO.

Then they measured levels of phenols in the cooked foods as well as in the raw foods.

Results: Frying and sautéing in olive oil yielded the most phenols in the finished dish—significantly increasing both the total amount and the healthful variety of these compounds. Boiling in water, or even water with a little olive oil added in, didn't increase phenols. It was the direct heating of veggies in olive oil that made the difference.

What's so great about phenols? These antioxidant compounds, found in many plant foods (fruits, vegetables, the olives that get turned into olive oil, even champagne) protect the body's cells against oxidation and inflammation that can promote chronic disease. People whose diets are rich in phenols are statistically less likely to develop heart disease, Alzheimer's disease and certain cancers.

How Olive Oil Makes Vegetables Even Healthier

To put the research in perspective, here are insights from registered dietitian Sharon Palmer, RDN…

One way that cooking in olive oil enhanced phenols in the study was that it helped make them easier to absorb. Other studies have also found that certain antioxidant compounds and nutrients in some vegetables become more bioavailable to your body in the presence of olive oil.

But some of the extra phenols in the cooked dishes came not from a change in the vegetables' phenols, but from additional phenols added from the olive oil itself. You'd get similar benefits from simply including EVOO in your diet—in your salad dressing, for example. You don't need to fry everything! Olive oil is rich in many phenolic compounds. A body of science backs up the benefits of eating a Mediterranean diet, which includes a generous dose of extra-virgin olive oil—in a diet filled with minimally processed foods such as grains, vegetables, fruits, legumes, herbs, nuts and seafood. In one major study, called PREDIMED, each increase of 10 grams a day in EVOO—about two teaspoons—was associated with a 10% reduction in risk for cardiovascular events.

What's so special about the golden nectar that is extra-virgin olive oil? Because extra-virgin olive oil is minimally processed, it retains many of those phenolic compounds present in the olive. And it is rich in heart-healthy monounsaturated fats. No wonder EVOO has been linked with many health bonuses, including reducing the risk for cardiovascular disease, improving the management of type 2 diabetes and even breast cancer prevention.

How much is enough? The PREDIMED Study found the most benefits related to consuming 57 grams—about four tablespoons—per day. So that means you can enjoy a little more than a tablespoon per meal drizzled over your foods as your source of additional fat.

The Formula for Vegetable Success

So, what's the best way to cook your vegetables with EVOO? Start with the real deal—extra-virgin olive oil—which works wonderfully in cooking methods as different as as sautéing, pan-frying, roasting or grilling. Don't fall for the myth that more is better. At 120 calories per tablespoon, EVOO is concentrated stuff. If you dump a quarter cup of it over your salad or pasta, you're adding an extra 480 calories to your meal, which most people simply can't afford. If you gain weight, that can quickly erase the potential health benefits from olive oil. The good news is that you don't need much olive oil to pump up both the flavor and healthfulness of your favorite vegetables.

When you're sautéing vegetables, for example, just heat one or two tablespoons of olive oil in a sauté pan or skillet and then add about four cups of any medley of vegetables. Drizzle a twist of lemon juice and your favorite pinch of spices and herbs, and sauté until just crisp-tender to make about four servings. One or two tablespoons is also a good amount for four servings when you're roasting vegetables or making a salad.

What about boiling vegetables in just a little water or steaming them? That's still nutritious—while it won't enhance their phenols, it actually retains nutrients such as vitamin C best—and you can make it more phenol-rich by simply tossing your steamed (or even microwaved) vegetables with a little EVOO.

Bottom line: It's fine to include some veggies sautéed or even fried in olive oil in your diet, but it's not the only way to get the health benefits of vegetables—or olive oil.

The Real Benefits of Mindful Eating

Study titled "Effects of a Mindfulness-Based Weight Loss Intervention in Adults with Obesity: A Randomized Clinical Trial" by researchers at University of California, San Francisco, et al., published in *Obesity*.

D oes "mindful eating" help you lose weight? That's what researchers at the University of California set out to find out. It is common knowledge that stress can lead to overeating, especially mindless eating when you're not even hungry. Stress is linked to weight gain, especially belly fat, plus increases in blood sugar and blood fats.

And it is also common knowledge that learning mindfulness helps people regulate their emotions, including eating habits, especially when they're stressed.

But whether mindfulness training actually helps people lose more weight than regular dieting hasn't been rigorously studied in a double-blind randomized controlled trial.

Until now. And there are indeed benefits to dieters—just not the ones that were expected.

Breathe Deeply, Feel Your Hunger

The California researchers studied about 200 obese men and women with an average age of 48. Participants didn't have diabetes, nor were they taking any medications that affected weight. About half of them entered into a standard weight-loss program for 16 weeks—healthy food choices leading to cutting calories by about 500 calories a day plus daily exercise such as walking and strength training. Once they completed the program, they were followed over the next 14 months.

The second group went through the same diet/exercise program but also worked with a trainer on mindfulness-based eating awareness, including meditation, with specific emphasis on becoming aware of the feelings of hunger, taste, cravings, emotions and other eating triggers.

Results...

•**The mindful dieters did lose a little more weight than the regular dieters**—more than one year after the study ended, they weighed about nine pounds less than at the beginning, compared to about five pounds less for the regular dieters. However, it wasn't statistically significant, which means it may have been due to chance.

•**Much more statistically significant were differences in cardio-metabolic health.** Fasting blood sugar for the regular dieters crept up about 4 mg/dl, but it dropped about 4 mg/dl for the mindful group.

•**Triglycerides**—blood fats associated with diabetes risk—went down for only the mindfulness group, too.

•**The triglyceride/HDL ratio,** an indicator of metabolic syndrome, which raises the risk for both heart disease and diabetes, improved only for the mindfulness group.

There was also a hint in the data that those who meditated the most lost the most weight and had the best improvements in health measurements. Interestingly, those who liked their mindfulness trainer—did better than those who didn't feel good about the trainer.

Bottom line? Mindfulness-based eating might help you lose a little extra weight. But even if it doesn't, there's a good chance that it'll make you significantly healthier.

Eight "Forever" Foods Every Healthy Kitchen Needs

Torey Armul, MS, RD, CSSD, a spokesperson for the Academy of Nutrition and Dietetics, counsels clients on sports nutrition, weight management and family/prenatal nutrition through her private practice in Columbus, Ohio. ToreyArmul.com

When are you most likely to order takeout food? If you're like many people, it's when you're low on groceries at home. Keep your cabinets and your freezer stocked with these eight staples, and you'll never be without a fast but healthy meal.

Frozen Shrimp

If you're out of fresh meat, you'll get a convenient protein-rich alternative with frozen shrimp. They're a good source of B vitamins and iron, which can help boost your metabolism and keep you feeling your best. Because of their smaller size, frozen shrimp also can be easier to cook and prepare than frozen beef, pork or chicken.

In fact, you can save yourself a step by buying precooked shrimp. That way you just need to reheat them and season as desired. Thaw the shrimp in a bowl of hot water for three to five minutes and remove the tails. Next, season with olive oil and dried herbs and spices, such as chipotle chili pepper, garlic powder or basil. Reheat for just a few minutes on the stovetop, in the oven or on the grill. Shrimp can be served by itself or added to rice, pasta, tortillas, tacos or salad.

Frozen Broccoli

Vegetables are one of the first foods to spoil in every grocery haul. Don't let that be a reason to skip your veggies! Fruits and vegetables should make up half of what we eat, although few Americans are meeting this recommended daily intake. Once your stash of fresh veggies runs out, frozen makes an excellent substitute. They are packaged at the peak of freshness, which means that they retain their nutritional content. Some frozen veggies taste more like fresh than others—that includes broccoli, which also is especially nutritious. Not a fan of broccoli? Always keep on hand frozen cauliflower, peas, green beans, asparagus, brussels sprouts or a frozen vegetable "medley" that you like.

Easy one-pot dinner: Add your favorite frozen vegetables to a pasta pot a few minutes before the pasta is finished cooking. (Don't worry, the vegetables won't make the pasta too cold.) Then drain the pasta and vegetables together and serve. Easy!

Tuna Packets

Tuna packets are another convenient source of protein, with the addition of heart-healthy omega-3 fats. They're ready in an instant, but unlike cans, they don't require draining (the nutritional content is similar to that of canned tuna, however). Packaged tuna has a long shelf life, making it a pantry prerequisite when your other options are limited.

Branch out from plain tuna with flavored tuna packets, such as lemon pepper, hot buffalo style, sweet and spicy (my favorite!) and sun-dried tomato and basil. They add taste and variety to your meal without adding too much additional sodium or calories. I use flavored tuna packets to spice up my usual sandwiches, salads and pasta dishes.

Canned Soup

Canned soup gets a bad rap for containing too much salt, fat, sugar, preservatives...or all of the above. I still recommend it because it can be a full, balanced meal. The trick is to buy only soups that aren't loaded with unhealthy ingredients. The best soups are broth- or vegetable-based (such as butternut squash, tomato, minestrone or chicken noodle) rather than cream-based. Look for soups labeled "low sodium," which means that they contain 140 mg or less of sodium per serving. "Reduced sodium" indicates only that the soup has less sodium than the original version, so it may not be low in salt after all. While you're comparing labels, choose the soup with less saturated fat (2 grams or less) and more fiber (2 grams or more) per serving.

You also can bulk up a can of soup by adding frozen vegetables, canned beans, leftover rice, packaged tuna or really any healthy food you have around.

Here's another kitchen hack: Canned soup makes a ready-made sauce. Some of my favorite soups to use as sauce are butternut squash, chunky tomato, Italian-style wedding and lentil vegetable. Just add the soup to cooked rice, pasta, quinoa, poultry or fish for a delicious sauce that's ready in seconds. Low-sodium varieties will help to moderate your daily sodium intake.

Canned Chickpeas

Beans are one of the most underrated foods at the store. They are cheap yet remarkably nutritious, loaded with plant-based protein and fiber. Chickpeas, also known as garbanzo beans, are an excellent source of iron, folate, phosphorus and manganese. They are exceptionally convenient and versatile. Eat them plain, with a dash of salt and pepper or mixed into your meal. Enjoy them warm or cold. Mash them to create a creamy hummuslike appetizer or to complement a main dish.

While you're stocking up on chickpeas, grab some canned lentils, black beans and kidney beans, too. They share a similar nutritional profile and can be seamlessly added to soups, salads, rice bowls, tacos and omelets.

Microwavable Rice

There is no faster meal-starter than a packet of microwavable rice. It's ready in just 90 seconds, and the brown and wild rice varieties are major sources of fiber. Rice is a healthy base for a variety of Asian and Mexican dishes, or it can add flavor and nutrition to traditional soups and salads. Should you worry about arsenic levels in rice? Not if you eat a variety of whole grains and practice good portion control.

You do pay for the convenience of microwavable rice, however. I wait for sales to stock up on the microwavable packages.

Whole-Wheat Pasta

Dried pasta will last for a year or more in your pantry, making it a healthy choice when you're out of fresher foods. It's ready in minutes and can be a delicious way to add nutrients to your meal. Most people think of pasta as a carbohydrate-rich indulgence rather than a nutritious meal choice. However, it all comes down to choosing the right kind and watching your portion size.

Buy 100% whole-wheat pasta—meaning that whole wheat is the only ingredient. It typically has a shelf life of one to two years. Whole-wheat pasta is an excellent source of fiber, which keeps your digestive tract healthy and running smoothly. It also contains a moderate amount of protein.

Typical pasta portions are way too large. Limit yourself to a healthy one-cup serving of cooked pasta, and add vegetables and beans to help fill you up.

Frozen Strawberries

Few foods are more perishable than fresh fruit. Luckily, frozen berries are a great alternative. One cup of frozen strawberries is low in calories but delivers 18% of your recommended daily fiber intake and 150% of your daily vitamin C. Like vegetables, fruit is frozen at its peak ripeness, preserving nutritional value.

Nosh on berries straight from the bag for a sweet and satisfying dessert (just give them a few minutes to thaw slightly). Want to sweeten up your breakfast with healthy antioxidants? Sauté frozen fruit in a saucepan for a berry sauce to drizzle over pancakes, yogurt and oatmeal. Strawberries also are great in smoothies and stirred into yogurt.

Save money when buying frozen fruit by waiting for sales, which usually happen when the fruit is in season. Diversify your choices with frozen mango, cherries, peaches and blueberries, all of which make a low-calorie dessert.

Have Your Green Veggies and Coumadin, Too

Timothy S. Harlan, MD, associate professor of medicine at the Tulane University School of Medicine in New Orleans. He is the author of *The Dr. Gourmet Diet for Coumadin Users* and *Vegetable Recipes for Coumadin Users*. Dr. Harlan is also executive director of the Goldring Center for Culinary Medicine, the world's first fully operational, full-time teaching kitchen at a medical school. DrGourmet.com

Could a spinach salad ever be considered dangerous? That may sound impossible. But if you're one of the millions of Americans who takes the popular blood thinner *warfarin* (Coumadin, Jantoven, Marevan, etc.) to help prevent stroke, heart attack or pulmonary embolism, chances are your doctor has told you to limit your intake of spinach and other vitamin K–rich foods.

It's true that vitamin K promotes blood clotting, and consuming too many foods that contain abundant amounts of this nutrient could weaken warfarin's effect.

Taken to the extreme, however, this dietary advice often causes warfarin users to become fearful of eating any of the highly nutritious foods that contain vitamin K.

What many people don't realize is that following this guideline too strictly creates almost as much of a problem as getting too much of this crucial nutrient, which has been shown to promote heart and bone health.

The solution: There is a simple way that you can have your warfarin—and your green veggies, too! *Here's how...*

The Stay-Safe Formula

If you watch TV, you've no doubt seen plenty of ads for the newer generation of blood thinners, such as *apixaban* (Eliquis), *rivaroxaban* (Xarelto) and *dabigatran* (Pradaxa). These medications work similarly to warfarin by blocking production of blood-clotting proteins in the body, but they use a different mechanism that doesn't require vitamin K vigilance.

Even though these newer blood-thinning drugs are being prescribed more and more, warfarin is still the most widely used medication for stroke and heart attack patients.

But the use of *warfarin* requires a delicate balancing act that weighs the risk for excessive bleeding against the risk for unwanted clotting. To keep tabs on how long it takes a patient's blood to clot, frequent blood testing is used (initially on a daily basis, then gradually decreased until a target level has been reached) to determine the patient's INR, which stands for "international normalized ratio." For most patients, the target for this standardized measurement ranges from about 2.0 to 3.0.

Other risks: In addition to the dietary considerations, warfarin interacts with a number of medications (such as certain antibiotics, other heart medications, cholesterol drugs and antidepressants) as well as supplements (including St. John's wort and ginkgo biloba).

Dr. Harlan's stay-safe formula: There is no definitive research pointing to optimal levels of vitamin K for warfarin users, but I find that most patients thrive on a plan in which their daily intake of this vitamin is about 75 micrograms (mcg) per day—a level that is lower than the recommended daily allowance for adults (90 mcg per day for women…and 120 mcg per day for men). That intake of vitamin K seems to strike the balance between offering an adequate amount of healthful foods rich in the vitamin while allowing warfarin to do its job.

A New Way to Eat Vitamin K

It's amazing to see how much the vitamin K content varies depending on the food. Some foods are absolute vitamin K powerhouses—one cup of raw parsley, for example, has a whopping 984 mcg…one cup of cooked spinach contains 888 mcg…and one cup of raw kale, 547 mcg.

Note: Cooking a vegetable will decrease its volume, but won't change the vitamin K content.

To avoid slipping into a vitamin K danger zone, I advise warfarin users to regularly incorporate vegetables with low-to-moderate amounts of vitamin K into their diet (up to 20 mcg per serving).

Good choices (serving sizes are one cup unless otherwise indicated): Arugula (one-half cup), beets, carrots, celery (one stalk), corn, eggplant, sweet red or green peppers, peas (one-half cup), turnips, tomatoes and zucchini.

Other foods that are naturally low in vitamin K include most fruits, cereals, grains, beans, seeds and tubers (such as white potatoes, sweet potatoes and yams).

A good rule of thumb: Stick to side dishes with 20 mcg to 25 mcg of vitamin K per serving and main courses with 35 mcg to 40 mcg per serving. That should keep you at a safe level.

But what if you reach your daily limit and are still craving some sautéed greens or a big kale salad? Don't despair. You can still enjoy these foods…as long as your intake of vitamin K is consistent.

This means that you can exceed 75 mcg of vitamin K per day—but you must consume the same amount of the vitamin every day. So you can have a spinach salad, but you need to eat the same-sized salad (or another dish with an equivalent amount of vitamin K) every single day.

Important: Be sure to first tell your doctor if you plan to increase your intake of vitamin K so that you can be closely monitored and, if needed, your dose of warfarin adjusted. The frequency of monitoring depends on the patient's specific circumstances.

To find the vitamin K content of various foods: Go to DrGourmet.com/md/warfarincomprehensive.pdf.

The "Safe" List

Unless you're a nutritionist, you probably don't know the vitamin K content of most foods off the top of your head. To help you stay safe when you're close to reaching your limit of the vitamin, here are some healthful foods that contain virtually no vitamin K in a single serving...

Acorn squash...raw mushrooms...cooked grits...yellow sweet pepper... cooked salmon, halibut or sole...cooked pork...light-meat turkey (no skin)... lemon, lime or orange...almonds...nonfat sour cream...rosemary, garlic powder or ground allspice, ginger or nutmeg.

What's the Perfect Diet? That Depends on You

Kristi Hughes, ND, naturopathic physician, director of medical education, Institute for Functional Medicine, Federal Way, Washington.

Margaret Mills, MS, functional nutrition clinical coordinator, Institue for Functional Medicine, Federal Way, Washington.

Mary Willis, RD, LD, CDE, nutrition services director, College Park Family Care Center, Overland Park, Kansas.

Paleo. Mediterranean. Vegetarian. High-protein. Low-carb. Gluten-free. Low-glycemic. Intermittent fasting. Organic. Probiotic. DASH. MIND. Detox. HELP!

If you want to eat in a healthier way to prevent or cure health problems, you have a dizzying number of choices. Unfortunately, those choices are confusing—and conflicting.

The truth is, no one diet is perfect for everyone. Some people have specific food sensitivities and respond well when they eliminate their "trigger" foods, while others do fine on a wide variety of healthy foods. Some thrive on moderate portions of high-carb whole foods, while others really need a low-carb approach. And so on.

What we really need are core principles for a healthy diet—and then ways to tailor them to our personal health needs. That is exactly what the Institute for Functional Medicine (IFM)—an organization that trains health professionals to treat the underlying causes of diseases—has developed. In a heroic attempt to bring clarity to the dietary "Tower of Babel," the IFM interviewed nutrition-oriented physicians, health-care practitioners and nutrition researchers and crossed-referenced the results with the scientific literature.

The good news: The IFM's Core Food Plan fits just about any healthy person's needs and is very customizable—in fact, it's designed to be customized. Read on to get the details of a healthy eating pattern that's good for nearly everyone—and ways you can work with a health professional to get it tailored for you.

An Evidence-Based Approach to a Healthy Diet

Why do we need a new way to eat? It's because in our society today, to a large extent, we don't eat real food. It's that simple. Add in our sedentary lifestyles, polluted environment and lack of sufficient sleep, and it's no wonder so many of us have high blood pressure, heart disease, diabetes, headaches and other chronic pain, chronic infections and too much body fat.

To break this cycle, the IFM's Core Food Plan can be a good place to start. IFM's director of medical education, Kristi Hughes, ND, emphasizes that it's not necessarily better than other well-established evidence-based dietary plans such as the Mediterranean Diet. Indeed, it derives some of its principles from that approach (as well as from Paleo). But the beauty of the Core Food Plan is that it provides dietary guidance that can be easily tailored to individual needs. And it does go a step beyond the official US dietary guidelines. For example, research suggests that consumption of high-glycemic grains and low-fat dairy, which are promoted by the US dietary guidelines, are not consistent with overall health. In contrast to those guidelines and most conventional nutrition advice, the IFM Core Food Plan emphasizes fresh whole foods with high phytonutrient diversity.

Nutritionist Mary Willis, RD, LD, CDE, who helped develop the Core Food Plan, says the challenge was to create a healthy eating plan that would help transition people away from the standard American diet (or what nutritionists fittingly call "SAD"). One key problem with SAD is the preponderance of highly-refined carbs with little or no nutritional value. Many people transitioning from SAD are consuming more than 50% of their calories from carbs, and most of those carbs are refined carbs from sugar and grains, not from vegetable or fruit sources.

The Core Food Plan, in contrast, is a balanced "plant-dominant" approach. It does include meat (if you want it to). But you can still think of Core as everything SAD isn't—high in vegetables (and fruits) from across the rainbow spectrum...low or moderately low in grain-based carbohydrates...low in sugar... and devoid of processed foods.

The Core Food Plan: What to Eat Every Day

The Core Food Plan is not a deprivation diet—in fact, it's actually pretty balanced when it comes to protein (25% of calories), fat (30%) and carbohydrates (45%). That all comes from nine distinct food groups (listed below). The appropriate servings are based on calorie needs and therapeutic considerations. To get an idea of what's included, consider the recommendations for the 1,800-to-2,200 calorie range, which is appropriate for an average man or a woman who is physically active. *Here's what you would eat each day...*

•**Proteins.** Seven or eight small "portions." This category, which includes animal and plant protein, is measured in "portions" rather than "servings." Each portion is small—just one ounce of meat, fish or poultry, one egg or one-half ounce of hard cheese, for example—but you can mix-and-match sources and have multiple portions at a meal. (A four-ounce filet mignon, for example, would be four portions.) The plan stresses "clean" sources of animal protein— lean, free-range, grass-fed, wild-caught. It can also be tailored to vegetarians— and vegans—with portions such as one ounce of tempeh or two ounces of firm tofu. When you eat your protein is an important factor. Americans do not eat enough high-quality protein at breakfast and/or lunch—and then overeat protein at dinner.

•**Legumes.** Two or three servings. One-half cup of cooked beans or lentils is one serving, so the total is one to one-and-a-half cups a day. Vegetarians and vegans, however, may want to increase their daily servings of legumes as a substitute for animal protein.

•**Dairy and dairy alternatives.** Three servings. Fermented dairy foods such as yogurt and kefir are emphasized over, say, milk, as they feed the "good" bacteria in the gut, which in turn help turn down inflammation. Nondairy alternatives such as almond and soy milk are also encouraged. One serving is eight ounces of milk or six ounces of Greek yogurt. In the Core Food Plan, "dairy" doesn't include cheese, which is in the protein category.

•**Nuts and seeds.** Three to five snack-sized servings.

Examples: 10 peanuts, six almonds, one tablespoon of sunflower seeds or one-half tablespoon of nut butter would each be considered one serving.

•**Fats and oils.** Four to five small servings. *Examples:* One teaspoon of butter or olive oil or two tablespoons of an oily food, such as avocado (one-eighth whole fruit). If you eat butter—which is considered a fat rather than a dairy food—choose butter made from the milk of grass-fed cows, which has a healthier balance of fats.

•**Nonstarchy vegetables.** 10 servings.

Example: One-half cup of cooked broccoli or spinach or one cup of salad greens. This is a big increase in veggies for many people. Most Americans get only two to four servings a day—and most are fried.

•**Starchy vegetables.** One or two servings.

Examples: One cup of cooked squash or one-half a medium potato.

•**Fruit.** Two or three servings.

Examples: One small apple, three-quarter cup of blueberries, one cup of melon. Including fruit in your diet provides antioxidants, fiber and key vitamins. The fiber blunts the body's response to sugar, so whole fruit, compared with foods with added sugars, is a lower-glycemic source of natural sweetness.

•**Grains.** Two servings.

Examples: One-third cup of cooked rice, one slice of bread. Grains are de-emphasized in the IFM food plans. Why? To make room for a robust amount of colorful plant foods from other food categories that are overlooked in the grain-dominant standard American diet. Americans put a bun or wrap or breading on everything! For people who need to avoid gluten, the IFM plan also includes many gluten-free grain picks including oats, quinoa, rice and millet.

The core plan emphasizes organic foods to reduce exposure to pesticides. It can be tailored to accommodate people who are avoiding gluten, dairy or animal foods. It can be customized for athletes, who may, for example, need extra protein. It can also be tailored for people who want to experiment with "intermittent fasting," which calls for certain very low-calorie days followed by normal eating days as a way to improve body composition, enhance metabolism and control weight.

Some people lose weight on the IFM Core Food Plan, but that's not the primary goal—or even the best measure of success. Rather, the emphasis is on improving health and maintaining a healthy way of eating for life. A person who transitions from SAD to Core can expect to have more energy, which in turn may motivate him or her to get more physically active. Those lifestyle changes could then lead to improvements in metabolic fitness and a reduced risk for chronic disease. Clinically, patients who switch to this eating style often report more focus and concentration, enhanced sleep, greater daily stamina and an improved sense of well-being.

If You Want to Try One of the IFM's Customized Food Plans...

While adopting the Core Food Plan itself would bring a world of improvement for many people, the IFM also has developed other plans to allow health professionals—including MDs, osteopaths, naturopaths, nutritionists, nurse practitioners and others—to help patients with specific, identified needs.

Some IFM plans are "first step" diets, while others are more advanced interventions for people with certain medical conditions. Some are designed to be short-term. As the IFM practitioner's guide states, "Nutritional and dietary needs may change or evolve as a patient moves through a layered healing process."

The first step interventions are...

•**Cardiometabolic Food Plan.** This is for people with cardiovascular and blood sugar–related issues such as insulin resistance and the problems that often go with them, including unhealthy cholesterol ratios, excess abdominal fat and high levels of inflammation. It emphasizes low-glycemic foods (which help keep blood sugar stable), increased fiber, meal timing and ideal serving sizes. Compared with the Core Food Plan, the macronutrient balance is slightly lower in carbohydrates and higher in protein—30% protein...30% fat...40% carbs.

•**Elimination Diet.** Pinpointing the foods causing food allergies, intolerances or sensitivities and eliminating them (and eventually reintroducing some) is the goal. According to the practitioner's guide, "Often, symptoms that have failed to respond to conventional medical therapy will resolve by following an elimination diet. After the initial period of eliminating foods, many chronic symptoms should improve or disappear."

One example of an advanced intervention is the Detox Food Plan, which builds on the Elimination Diet by eliminating certain trigger foods but then goes a step further by emphasizing avoidance of environmental toxins (in plastics for example), consumption of organic foods and consumption of specific therapeutic foods that support the gut, liver and kidneys. These emphasize cruciferous vegetables such as broccoli and cauliflower, dark leafy greens and bitter greens, for example.

There are also customizable "GI specific dietary interventions" for people with gastrointestinal complaints who have followed the elimination diet but are still experiencing symptoms. They include an antifungal (anti-Candida) diet, a low-FODMAP diet and others. The Mito Food Plan ("Mito" is short for mitochondria, the "energy factories" inside each cell) is designed to nutritionally support people with pain and fatigue syndromes as well as those who are at risk for autoimmune conditions or those experiencing neurological concerns. It is a strict anti-inflammatory, low-glycemic, gluten-free, low-grain, high-quality-fats approach to eating. There's also a ReNew Food Plan, which can be used as a modified elimination diet and is designed to be "a whole systems reboot and system detox." It's geared toward people with autoimmune, gastrointestinal, neurological and other chronic health conditions. It eliminates sugar, dairy, grains (including gluten-free), alcohol, caffeine, artificial sweeteners, processed foods that contain heavy metals and foods high in pro-inflammatory saturated animal fats.

Do these customized versions really work? To be clear, they have not been studied in clinical trials but rather are based on clinical practice in functional medicine and related nutrition research. Various research projects are in the works—the Cleveland Clinic, for example, collaborated in the creation of the ReNew plan and is using it with some of its patients. The Cleveland Clinic is also using the Mito plan for certain patients of the clinic's Center for Functional Medicine.

While the Core Food Plan is fine for anyone who's generally healthy, the more personalized and specific versions are really designed to be undertaken with the supervision of a medical professional, nutrition professional or functional medicine health coach trained to customize the food plan to the individual. To find a health-care professional who is trained in the IFM approach, go to FunctionalMedicine.org and choose "find a practitioner." Additionally, the Functional Medicine Coaching Academy trains health coaches in collaboration with the IFM, and you may be able to find a nutrition coach through it.

The Hidden Danger in Your Food: How It's Cooked May Increase Your Risk for Chronic Illness

Sandra Woodruff, RD, a registered dietitian and nutrition consultant based in Tallahassee, Florida. **Helen Vlassara, MD,** an endocrinologist and professor at Mount Sinai School of Medicine in New York City, where she directs the Experimental Diabetes and Aging Division. They are coauthors of *The AGE-Less Way: Escape America's Overeating Epidemic.* TheAGE-lessWay.com

Some of the most serious chronic health problems in the US, including Alzheimer's disease, cancer, diabetes and kidney and heart disease, have been linked to what we eat—processed foods, fast food, red meat, etc. What may surprise you is that the increased health risks from these foods may be due in large part to how they are cooked.

Dry-heat cooking, such as grilling, broiling, frying and even baking and roasting, greatly increases levels of advanced glycation end-products (AGEs), also known as glycotoxins. Small amounts of these chemical compounds are naturally present in all foods, but their levels rise dramatically when foods are subjected to dry heat, which frequently occurs both in home cooking and in commercial food preparation.

The danger: AGEs are oxidants that produce free radicals, damage DNA, trigger inflammation throughout the body and accelerate the aging process. They also make cholesterol more likely to cling to artery walls, the underlying cause of most heart attacks. Some researchers now believe that AGEs can be linked to most chronic diseases.

A New Threat

A century ago, people mainly ate fresh, homemade foods, such as grains, vegetables, legumes and fruits, with relatively small amounts of meat. The processed food industry was still in its infancy.

However, in the following decades, meat portions grew larger, and Americans acquired a strong desire for the intense flavors, aromas and colors in commercially prepared "browned" foods, such as crackers, chips, cookies, grilled and broiled meats, french fries, pizza, etc. During this time, the rates of heart disease, diabetes and other chronic diseases started to rise. This wasn't a coincidence—the rich taste, smell and appearance of these foods primarily come from AGEs.

Our bodies can neutralize the small amounts of AGEs that are naturally found in foods (and that we produce as a by-product of metabolism). But our defense mechanisms are overwhelmed with the high amounts that are now very common in the typical American diet.

How Much Is Too Much?

AGEs are measured in kilounits (kU). We recommend consuming no more than 5,000 kU to 8,000 kU per day. Recent studies have shown that the average American typically consumes more than 15,000 kU daily, and many people eat well over 20,000 kU daily.

Reducing dietary AGEs may be especially important for people with diabetes because high blood sugar levels cause more AGEs to form. It's also crucial for people with kidney disease because they are less able to remove AGEs from the body. AGEs also are elevated in patients with heart disease, obesity and dementia.

Researchers can measure the amounts of AGEs in the blood, but doctors don't commonly use this test because it's not currently available for commercial use. What your doctor can do is measure levels of C-reactive protein (CRP), a marker for inflammation. If your level is high (above 3 mg/dL), you may have excessive AGEs in your blood. If you eat a lot of grilled, broiled and roasted meats, for example, and/or heat-treated processed foods, this also means your AGE levels are likely too high.

An "AGE-Less" Diet

Our studies have shown that people who make simple dietary changes can reduce their levels of AGEs by more than 50% in four months. The reduction is accompanied by a similar decrease in CRP levels. *Helpful strategies...*

•**Eat less animal protein.** Animal protein, especially red meat, is among the main sources of AGEs—and the levels can multiply tenfold when the meat is grilled, broiled, baked or roasted. Helpful: Eat beef no more than three times a week.

Because animal fat also contributes to AGE intake, eat lean meats. They have fewer AGEs than higher-fat meats. Animal fats such as butter also are higher in AGEs than plant fats such as olive oil.

Best approach: Fill three-quarters of your plate with plant foods, such as vegetables, whole grains, legumes and fruits, and leave no more than one-quarter of the plate for animal foods, such as meats and cheeses.

• **Soups and stews are tasty ways to serve small portions of meat.** Also enjoy more meatless meals, such as vegetarian chili or veggie burgers. Nonfat milk and yogurt are low in AGEs and are a good way to add protein to meals and snacks.

• **Avoid dry-heat cooking, such as grilling, broiling, baking, roasting and frying.** High, dry heat greatly increases AGEs. Example: A piece of raw meat might have 500 kU to 700 kU of AGEs. But after the meat is broiled, the level can rise to 5,000 kU to 8,000 kU.

Better approach: Cook with moist heat—stew, poach, steam, boil or microwave. A piece of chicken that's poached or boiled, for example, will have about 1,000 kU. The same piece of chicken will have about 5,000 kU when it's broiled.

If you have a desire for grilled or roasted foods, vegetables and fruits are better choices than meats. These foods have far fewer AGEs than meats and fats when cooked with dry heat.

If you do cook with dry heat, marinate first. The eventual formation of AGEs is reduced by about 50% when raw meats are marinated in acidic ingredients, such as vinegar or lemon juice. For each pound of meat, use the juice from two lemons or an equivalent amount of vinegar or lime juice plus enough water to cover the meat (about one cup). Add some garlic and/or herbs for extra flavor. Avoid commercial marinades since they're usually high in sugar and/or oil, which will increase AGEs.

• **Reheat gently.** Microwaving is a good method for reheating meats and other foods. Be sure to include plenty of liquid and reheat to a safe temperature to prevent the possibility of food-borne illness due, for example, to E. coli or salmonella.

Soups, sauces and gravies should be brought to a boil. Leftovers such as meats and casseroles should be reheated to 165°F.

• **Don't eat certain foods together.** Consuming meats with foods that are high in sugar—for example, having a slice of cake after eating a hamburger—allows existing AGEs in the meat to interact with the sugars in the cake, creating higher levels of AGEs. Similarly, eating meats with very high-fat foods, such as a hamburger topped with bacon and cheese, will produce far more AGEs than consuming these foods by themselves.

•**Focus on fresh foods.** Because processed foods have high levels of AGEs, fresh foods and foods that have been minimally processed are a much better choice.

A serving of rice, for example, will have almost no AGEs, but the same amount of crispy rice cereal will have 600 kU. Avoid takeout and convenience foods, such as fast-food burgers, fries and pizza.

Warning: Any food that has been browned or crisped, such as cookies, crackers, chips, etc., will be high in AGEs.

If you're having a hard time sorting out or applying the findings of nutrition or weight-loss studies to your life, aren't getting the promised benefits of the latest superfood, or just aren't sure how to get the most health out of food and still enjoy eating (yes, kale has its limits!), an experienced nutrition coach can help. In fact, no matter what your goals—lower weight, more energy, fewer chaotic meals, clearer thinking, less illness, etc.—if you're stuck in second gear or sliding into reverse, a good coach can identify why you're not making progress and help you get around the roadblocks.

But first you have to find the right specialist. Not all people who call themselves nutrition, diet or health coaches have the same training and knowledge about nutrition. While you may not find every type of credentialed nutrition coach in your area, look for a registered dietitian (RD) or registered dietitian nutritionist (RDN), pros who must have at least a bachelor's degree with courses in dietetics and must work in a supervised internship before taking a certification exam from the Commission on Dietetic Registration of the Academy of Nutrition and Dietetics. If there are no RDs or RDNs practicing near you, all states and the District of Columbia—except for Arizona, Colorado, Michigan and New Jersey—have requirements for either a licensed dietitian nutritionist (LDN) or certified dietitian nutritionist (CDN), who will have met the specific requirements of the particular state.

Be aware that some credentials sound alike but are actually very different: A certified nutrition specialist (CNS) has an extensive level of training—a master's degree or doctorate, 1,000 hours of supervised experience and the deepest level of knowledge, often in specialty areas such as therapeutic nutrition, helpful for someone with a chronic condition or a patient in the hospital. On the other hand, all that's required to be a certified nutrition consultant (CNC) is a high school degree and passing grades on less than a dozen open-book tests.

Nutritional counseling may be covered by your health insurance company if it deems the service medically necessary and you choose a licensed nutritionist, RD, or nurse with nutrition training (check your policy for specifics). Medicare offers nutrition therapy coverage when ordered by your doctor. But even if you have to dip into your own pocket to hire someone, the advice and training you get may be worth every penny in terms of feeling better and getting healthier.

Is Healthy Eating a Puzzle? A Nutrition Coach Can Solve It!

Nicole Patience, RD, LDN, CDE, CEDRD, a registered dietitian, licensed dietitian nutritionist, certified diabetes educator, and certified eating disorders registered dietitian at Joslin Diabetes Center in Boston.

If you have a specific medical problem, a coach who also has condition-specific qualifications may be able to help you even more. *Here are some examples…*

If you have diabetes: A RD who's also a certified diabetes educator (CDE) can show you ways to better control blood sugar and craft a nutritious diet that includes your favorite foods. Diabetes educators keep up with the latest health guidelines including diabetes drugs and their interactions with food—vital information for people with the condition. They also understand heart health, high blood pressure and many health problems that people with diabetes often face.

If you have cancer: A dietitian who specializes in oncology nutrition (a board-certified specialist in oncology nutrition or CSO) can help you choose the most nutritious foods during treatment and recovery and help you manage treatment side effects ranging from fatigue to taste changes.

If you have an eating disorder: Some RDs are also credentialed as certified eating disorders registered dietitians or CEDRDs. A CEDRD can help you rebuild a healthy relationship with food, showing you how to move beyond the extensive rules, habits or rituals around food you may have developed.

Be Sure to Voice Your Goals

Honestly communicating your personal goals and your food stumbling blocks with your coach is essential. Do you want to run a half-marathon or find ways to cook more healthful meals on a time-and-money budget? *The more specifics you can share with your coach, the better he/she can help you…*

•**Your past experience with dieting.** Detail what worked or didn't work, including any aspects of diets that you found easy or hard to maintain.

•**Your food likes and dislikes.** Perhaps you love chicken, pasta and green veggies like spinach, but you dislike pork, shellfish, mushrooms and anything with garlic. Knowing your likes and dislikes gives your coach a place to start. (Don't try to make yourself sound less picky than you are—your coach is there to help the real you!)

•**Your health.** Reveal any allergies or other health problems you have that pose diet restrictions. Mention any supplements (including vitamins) and medications that you take. Some can negatively interact with certain foods.

•**Your activity level.** Are you sedentary, moderately active or very active? Be honest! How much you move goes into determining how much fuel you need to reach your goals.

•**Cultural or religious influences on food choices.** Share if beef, pork or shellfish is off-limits, for example.

•**Your food budget.** Healthy food doesn't have to be expensive food. Discuss how much of your paycheck can go to groceries. If money is tight, your coach can give you the budget-friendly food choices you can make.

•**Your comfort level with cooking.** If you want to do more cooking from scratch, your coach may match recipes to your skill level, teach you new techniques or suggest podcasts, blogs or videos for ideas to inspire you and help you feel more confident. If you eat out a lot or rely on prepared foods, he can suggest the best choices from your favorite menus.

•**Your comfort foods.** You won't stick to a plan if all your favorites are left out! But your coach can show you clever ways to find a healthier balance and feel satisfied from your meals. For example, if vegetables are a scarcity at dinner now, this might include creative ways to add volume with vegetables that pair well with the main protein.

•**How easy it is for you to food shop.** If your work schedule or physical condition makes this difficult, your coach may suggest an online food service that delivers or offers a pick-up on your way home.

•**Your particular challenges.** Maybe you eat well at breakfast and dinner, but lunches are usually a slice of pizza or a fast-food burger because that's all you think you have time for. Your coach can give you workable ideas for getting over your own personal humps in ways you might not have considered.

With all of the above information, your coach can put together a customized, flexible and realistic plan for you both at home and on the go.

Index